"A very fine piece of work, opening up how Moore's erotic life was able to unfold in her analysis. Delicately and at the same time passionately told, this is a valuable picture into therapy from an analysand's experience."

Susie Orbach, author of *Fat is a Feminist Issue* (1978), *The Impossibility of Sex* (2000) and ten other books on psychoanalysis; Fellow of the Royal Society of Literature; and recipient of Lifetime Achievement Award from the British Psychoanalytic Society

"This is an impressive book by Frances Moore. With an authoritative voice she gives an honest account of the patient's experience of the frustrations and the benefits of the erotic transference in psychotherapy. With a rare and valuable insight from the patient's point of view she gives both a lively and a well-researched expression of the therapeutic process as it is lived and understood."

David Mann, author of *Psychotherapy – An Erotic Relationship: Transference and Countertransference Passions* (1997); editor of *Erotic Transference and Countertransference: Clinical Practice in Psychotherapy* (1999) and *Love and Hate: Psychoanalytic Perspectives* (2002); and psychoanalytic psychotherapist in Tunbridge Wells

"This is a story of the ever-present erotic dimension of analysis and how it transforms and intensifies lived experience. Though a layperson – thankfully! – Moore wrestles with complicated themes, e.g., how different forms of erotic transferences can defend against one another, coexist (background sensuality and sexual desire) and ultimately promote growth. With precise and truthful articulation, Moore describes erotic love as the basis of elemental passions and human core vitality.

This is a story of how a woman becomes receptive to her own potency, learning to harness her power and beauty. Through her eyes, we also experience a calm and unafraid analyst willing to go the distance. Anyone doubting the usefulness of erotic transferences as an essential transformational power should read this book."

Andrea Celenza, author of *Erotic Revelations* (2014), *Sexual Boundary Violations* (2007) and *Transference, Love, Being: Essential Essays from the Field* (2022); training and supervising analyst, Boston Psychoanalytic Society and Institute

Growing Through the Erotic Transference

The book offers an in-depth case study of the erotic transference experienced by a female analysand with her male analyst, exploring how the shifting phases of erotic transference help the analysand to understand, rediscover and redefine herself with transformative growth.

The first half of the book tells the story of the analysis, which is richly imbued with the erotic from the beginning. It describes the complexity of the relationship between analyst and analysand and how the patient is able to grow through experiencing, analysing and progressing through the erotic transference. The second half of the book consists of five reflections, highlighting relative blind spots in the current thinking on the erotic transference and counter-transference. The author explores the dynamics of power, potency and erotic turn-on between male analyst and female analysand and considers the implications for the erotic transference when the patient is a sexual abuse survivor. She also explores the nature of 'transference love' itself: whether it is 'real love' and how both members of the dyad can surrender to it enough to grow, while not losing their bearings. The final reflection considers the role of the patient's voice in the psychoanalytic literature and argues the need for more of such accounts to enrich our understanding of this vital area.

Writing as the patient, the author is able to share a remarkable, frank and revealing glimpse into their personal experience of analysis, making this book essential reading for psychoanalysts, psychotherapists and anyone interested in understanding analysis in more depth.

Frances H. Moore first graduated as a performing musician from one of the major music conservatoires before gaining a Masters and a PhD in Anthropology of Music as a scholar at an Ivy League University. Her first published academic book is based on this PhD.

After transitioning to work in International Business, she completed an Executive MBA. She now specialises in leadership development, culture change and engagement strategies for international organisations going through major transformations. She has lived on three continents and has worked in over 20 countries.

Moore is passionate about helping others grow and find their full voices – in particular, girls and women. She was a volunteer teacher for a year in Africa and continues to mentor and train for young people's organisations. She was founding trustee/executive board member for two women's charities. She has written and published three children's books with brave, strong girl characters to counteract the passive princess stereotypes of the traditional tales.

In the wake of her own marriage breakdown, the 'quest for voice' became deeply personal. As an analysand, she immersed herself in the experience of analysis and voraciously absorbed the psychoanalytic literature as she followed her own transformative path. Her powerful experiences of the erotic transference are chronicled in this book.

The author is publishing this book under an adjusted name, to respect the privacy of her family.

Routledge Focus on Mental Health

Routledge Focus on Mental Health presents short books on current topics, linking in with cutting-edge research and practice.

Titles in the series:

For a full list of titles in this series, please visit www.routledge.com/ Routledge-Focus-on-Mental-Health/book-series/RFMH.

Growing Through the Erotic Transference

An Analysand's Journey

Frances H. Moore

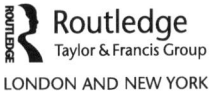

Routledge
Taylor & Francis Group

LONDON AND NEW YORK

First published 2023
by Routledge
4 Park Square, Milton Park, Abingdon, Oxon OX14 4RN

and by Routledge
605 Third Avenue, New York, NY 10158

Routledge is an imprint of the Taylor & Francis Group, an informa business

British Library Cataloguing-in-Publication Data
A catalogue record for this book is available from the British Library

Library of Congress Cataloging-in-Publication Data
Names: Moore, Frances H. (Pseudonym), author.
Title: Growing through the erotic transference : an analysand's journey /
    Frances H. Moore.
Description: Abingdon, Oxon ; New York, NY : Routledge, 2023. | Includes
    bibliographical references and index.
Identifiers: LCCN 2022020118 (print) | LCCN 2022020119 (ebook) |
    ISBN 9781032353982 (hardback) | ISBN 9781032353999 (paperback) |
    ISBN 9781003326700 (ebook)
Subjects: LCSH: Moore, Frances H. (Pseudonym)—Mental health. |
    Psychotherapy—Erotic aspects—Case studies. | Transference
    (Psychology)—Case studies. | Countertransference (Psychology)—
    Case studies. | Psychotherapist and patient—Case studies. | Women
    analysands—Biography.
Classification: LCC RC489.E75 M66 2023 (print) | LCC RC489.E75
    (ebook) | DDC 616.89/14—dc23/eng/20220601
LC record available at https://lccn.loc.gov/2022020118
LC ebook record available at https://lccn.loc.gov/2022020119

ISBN: 978-1-032-35398-2 (hbk)
ISBN: 978-1-032-35399-9 (pbk)
ISBN: 978-1-003-32670-0 (ebk)

DOI: 10.4324/9781003326700

Typeset in Times New Roman
by Apex CoVantage, LLC

To my loved ones, who made me who I am.

To the power of excellent, high-integrity psychoanalysis, which made me even better.

And to women and girls, in their quest to find themselves and their voices.

Contents

Introduction

Growing through the erotic transference

Writing this book has been invigorating. The working through and daring to express makes one tingle rather. It pales in comparison, though, to the effects of the erotic in the consulting room.

For me, as a woman patient working with a male analyst, the erotic transference was no static feeling, but rather a series of emotions and sensations pulling me through the stages of seduction, penetration and birth. It then threw me into the crashing paternal transference – highly unsettling in its tone of erotic fear – before cradling me in the maternal, couched in the soft sensuality of my own body. All this had to be experienced before desire, the most traditional form of the erotic transference, could be unleashed. Throughout, I was gradually reparented by my analyst, as he stayed next to me through all these journeys. I grew by noticing, grappling with, surrendering to and reshaping the shifting strands and tones of erotic love and aggression experienced via the transference. I learned about myself and confronted fundamental fears that I hadn't known I had by observing how I responded to the intimacy my analyst offered: always held exquisitely by him within its proper frame.

What do we mean by the erotic? I won't belabour my definition; it's in my nature to rebel against the overly theoretical. I prefer to embrace the lived reality of sex and the sexual, to write in a clear enough way for non-experts like myself to understand and to avoid dulling the felt experience of analysis that forms the foundation of progress for the patient. In this spirit, I focus here on telling a story; you will find no comprehensive literature review and little grappling with the more theoretical framings of the field. Long words I use are more likely to be "rapturous" or "voluptuous" than "Kleinian" or "pre-Oedipal", and I have kept my more theoretical meanderings to the footnotes and reflections section.

So, the word erotic, for me, simply includes the patient's full range of bodily, sexual and sensual understanding of themselves and their relating to

DOI: 10.4324/9781003326700-1

others, with the erotic transference being any of these which use the analyst as the vehicle for experience.

The erotic transference was originally viewed as a form of resistance (Freud 1915). Indeed, it can stop an analysis in its tracks if mishandled or if the patient refuses to reflect upon their feelings. Certainly, when it is viewed merely as a question of whether the patient feels attraction to the therapist, there is little that is creative about it. Yet, texts of the last 35 years have presented a more enriching view of the erotic and its role in the consulting room. The most seminal include: Gorkin (1985), Davies (1994), Wrye and Welles (1994), Mann (1997 and 1999), Maroda (1999), Orbach (2000), Schaverian (2006), Celenza (2014, 2023) and Atlas (2016). While arguing gently amongst themselves, these analysts all recognise that the dyad's willingness to experience and explore the erotic within the proper frame can help a patient understand themselves and even transform.

David Mann (1997, 9–10) perhaps expresses it best:

> Through the erotic, light is shone on the deepest recesses of the psyche. . . . The heart of the unconscious is visible in all its elemental passion and in so opening, allows for the prospect of transformation and psychic growth.

By remaining receptive and present with the patient, then, much fine work can be achieved. Love, in all its psychological forms, must definitely be on the agenda.

And so must erotic fear and aggression. The more desire-driven aspects of the love transference (the classic challenge of the patient 'falling in love') are more prominent in the literature, starting with Freud's own seminal note (1915). Equally or more important is the fear-driven erotic transference, fuelled by memories of abuse or by the lesser boundary violations many of us experience in childhood. This seems far less discussed, perhaps because it is less palatable for analysts to grapple with. This book explores both head on.

Despite its rich potential for transformation, the erotic is a challenging territory for both analysts and analysands to navigate; in Spector-Person's words, it is "both a goldmine and minefield" (1985, 163). Quite simply, it can go horribly wrong – most acutely when an analyst abuses their patient,[1] but also in many subtler forms of mismanagement. Considering how fraught with danger it is (and perhaps because of this), I believe we still lack sufficient support and insight. In Balsam's (2012, 4) words, "by our own theory of repression, this group collusion, and the resulting neglect, are markers not of insignificance, but of a vital import that we have yet to understand".[2]

My hope is that this book helps to contribute to deeper understanding by providing one additional lens from which analysts can consider their own work with the erotic. It tells the story of one successful navigation of the territory, sharing my understanding of the progressive phases of erotic transference through the first 2 years of my own analysis. You will hear my voice evolve through this journey; I have resisted unifying the tone or drawing conclusions about a phase based on self-discoveries that came later. In this, I hope to mirror the relatively visceral, 'unfolding' experience of the actual consulting room.

I conclude with 5 'reflection' chapters, further exploring the erotic dynamic between male analyst and female analysand. I focus on areas which I find both evocative and relatively neglected in the literature. I offer these reflections as provocations – as a springboard for discussion, rather than a manifesto.[3] First, I discuss the dynamics of power between male analysts and female analysands and the relationship between gratitude, suffering and turn-on. Second, I consider the relative neglect of the fear-based erotic transference and what I believe is an over-emphasis on resistance. I then consider the specific needs and sensitivities around the erotic transference for victims of abuse and boundary violation. The fourth reflection is on the nature of transference love itself: is it real love, and how can both members of the dyad surrender to it enough to grow without losing their bearings? My final reflection considers the role of the patient's voice in the psychoanalytic literature. For along with offering an in-depth case study, this book is unusual in being written by a lay patient. I consider the importance of this patient voice and argue the need for more such accounts in closing.

Before we begin, though, it is worth pausing on this question of voice: first, from the point of view of naming. Talking about patients has always been tricky for psychoanalysis. Pseudonyms, the changing of biographical details, merged or semi-fictitious 'illustrative' case studies are just some of the necessary techniques used to protect patients' confidentiality. Yet there are also downsides to these approaches. They can feel dehumanising for patients or even imply there is reason for shame. They also limit the depth and verity of case studies that the field can learn from.

As the patient in this case study, I am freer to share my own story. I feel able to because my analysis left me with a liberating lack of shame: a willingness to be heard and seen. Yet as most readers will know, the liberation we gain from therapy must always reconcile itself with the external world. Considering the delicacy of the topic and that my family are included in these pages, I wanted to respect their privacy. For this reason, I have published this book under an adjusted name: very close to my own, but not so easily linked to me on the internet.

As the patient in the case study, my voice is unusual. No one can recount my experiences of my analysis as fully. I have a PhD in the humanities and have absorbed a range of the psychoanalytic literature. By writing as the patient, I offer a rare female voice in the exploration of the male analyst-female analysand dyad. In all these senses, I can bring a rich perspective. Yet my voice is inevitably different from those who have been trained in the field and whose framing of issues have been honed through thousands of hours of practice and through membership within the analytic community. One could view this fresh perspective either as uninformed or uncorrupted!

How much input has my analyst had in this book? In some ways, the answer is quite simple; while he has contributed greatly to my growth, he has offered no input into the writing or editing of this book. While we talked about what my writing meant to me, I don't know whether he agrees with my interpretations of what happened; he always steered clear of explicitly theoretical interpretations within sessions, for which I am grateful. Thus, the authorial voice is mine, as are the interpretations and inevitable misinterpretations of what happened between us.

Nevertheless, we co-produced the analysis from which this book is born. One could view this as its own story of erotic coupling. Atlas (2016, 23) captures some of this complexity when exploring the ownership of the case studies she has written: "I do not believe we can definitely know what belongs to us and what belongs to our patients; our minds are interwoven, project and interject, and our narratives are co-created . . . parallel and counter-transferential processes abound".

I thank my analyst for this interweaving: for the gift of this journey and this book, which could not exist without him.

And now, my friends, the story.

Notes

1 Across decades, research has consistently indicated that around 5–12% of heterosexual male therapists have acted out sexually with their female patients. Celenza (2007) offers the most comprehensive review and consideration of this issue. For further detail, see: Pope, Keith-Spiegel and Tabachnick (1986), Rutter (1989), Carr and Robinson (1990), Jehu (1994), Celenza and Gabbard (2003), and Springer (2006).

2 Balsam refers here to the neglect of women's bodies, in particular of childbirth, within psychoanalytic discussion.

3 The reflections are, of course, limited by my own experience, and I fully acknowledge the rich and diverse aspects of the erotic transference they fail to touch upon. For example, I have focussed almost exclusively on the male analyst-female analysand dyad. There is extensive, rich work – particularly by women analysts – on different gender configurations, including: Orbach (2000), McDougall (1995), Schaverian (2006), Celenza (2014), Maroda (1999). As a white, middle class,

educated, economically comfortable woman working with a therapist of similar demographic, I have had the privilege of treating race and socio-economic factors as a relatively invisible part of these discussions. Neither have I touched on any LGBTQIA+ dynamics. These framings are equally important, valid and rich; I simply lack the qualifications and experience to comment on them.

References

Atlas, G. (2016) *The Enigma of Desire, Sex, Longing, and Belonging in Psychoanalysis*. New York and London: Routledge.

Balsam, R. (2012) *Women's Bodies in Psychoanalysis*. New York: Routledge.

Beard, M. (2017) *Women & Power: A Manifesto*. London: Profile Books.

Carr, M. and Robinson, G. (1990) 'Fatal attraction: The ethical and clinical dilemma of patient-therapist sex'. In *Canada Journal of Psychiat*, 35: 122–127.

Celenza, A. (2007) *Sexual Boundary Violations: Therapeutic, Supervisory, and Academic Contexts*. New York: Aronson.

Celenza, A. (2014) *Erotic Revelations, Clinical Applications and Perverse Scenarios*. New York: Routledge.

Celenza, A. (2023) *Transference, Love, Being: Essential Essays from the Field*. New York: Routledge.

Celenza, A. and Gabbard, G.O. (2003) 'Analysts who commit sexual boundary violations: A lost cause?' In *Journal of the American Pscyhoanalytic Association*, 51(2), 617–636.

Davies, J. M. (1994) 'Love in the afternoon: A relationship reconsideration of desire and dread in the countertransference.' In *Psychoanalytic Dialogues*, 4, 153–170.

Freud, S. (1915) 'Observations on transference love', in *Standard Edition Vol. 12*. London: Hogarth Press.

Gorkin, M. (1985) 'Varieties of sexualised Countertransference.' In *Pyschoanalytic Review*, 72(3), 421–440.

Jehu, D. (1994) *Patients as Victims: Sexual Abuse in Psychotherapy and Counselling*. London: John Wiley & Sons.

Mann, D. (1997) *Psychotherapy: An Erotic Relationship. Transference and Countertransference Passions*. New York: Routledge.

Mann, D. (ed.) (1999) *Erotic Transference and Counter-Transference*. London: Routledge.

Maroda, K. (1999) *Seduction, Surrender, and Transformation: Emotional Engagement in the Analytic Process*. London: The Analytic Press.

McDougall, J. (1995) *The Many Faces of Eros: A Psychoanalytic Exploration of Human Sexuality*. London: Free Association Press.

Orbach, S. (2000) *The Impossibility of Sex*. New York: Touchstone.

Pope, K., Keith-Spiegel, P. and Tabachnick, B. (1986) 'Sexual attraction to clients: The human therapist and the (sometimes) inhuman training systems.' In *American Psychologist*, 41, 147–158.

Rutter, M.P. (1989) *Sex in the Forbidden Zone*. London: Mandala.

Schaverian, J. (ed.) (2006). *Gender, Countertransference and the Erotic Transference: Perspectives from Analytical Psychology and Psychoanalysis*. London and New York: Routledge.

Spector-Person, E. (1985) 'The erotic transference in women and men: Differences and consequences.' In *Journal of the American Academy of Psychoanalysis*, 13, 159–180.

Springer, A. (2006). 'Paying homage to the power of love', in *Gender, Countertransference and the Erotic Transference: Perspectives from Analytical Psychology and Psychoanalysis*. London and New York: Routledge.

Wrye, H.K. and Welles, J.K. (1994) *The Narration of Desire: Erotic Transferences and Countertransferences*. Hillsdale, NJ: Analytic Press.

Part 1
The story

Meeting

"A safe landing place"

I began with three joint sessions with my then-husband. We came far too late to be helped, and by the second session (a month before our child's sixth birthday), I decided to end the marriage, as my husband was in love with and failing to give up a much younger woman. I had been with him since I was 17; 21 years, which was 2 years less than the age of his new partner. He was the only man I had ever been with, and I had remained very much in love. It had been a tranquil, apparently happy marriage until the cataclysm of revealed truths just 3 months earlier. In the third session, my husband confirmed he was happy for me to continue to see our analyst on my own (he had his own individual therapist in place). Thus, he handed me over to another man and exited stage left.

This man provided me with a safe landing place as I struggled through the grief. I was struck by his reticence and his ability to notice things I could not. I took to therapy intensely and soon found myself enlivened with a sense of adventure and new discovery. Within a month, I was speaking to my analyst in my head and thinking about my therapy constantly. In addition to helping me process my grief, it gave me a focus and energy – an aliveness I badly needed to ease the desolation of my husband's departure. It felt a lot like falling in love, but with transformation and self-discovery *through* him, rather than *with* him (I told myself).

DOI: 10.4324/9781003326700-3

Testing power and potency

"Ors can be ands"

"There is something masculine about you" was my husband's explanation for why he was unfaithful and why he would not contemplate reigniting our physical life. With this simple sentence, my husband struck at two things simultaneously. On a personal level, he amplified a hurt that lay beneath the more explicit pain of his infidelity – that as a woman, I was somehow inadequate. Second, he unthinkingly evoked century-old psychoanalytic concepts (and indeed more widely socially embedded doctrines) of what women should and should not be.

I have long hair, and my body is soft and curvaceous. I am also softly spoken, prefer listening to talking and spend a large proportion of my time caring for other people's needs. Yet if men alone are meant to be proactive, empowered, independent, strategic-minded, decisive, intellectual and high-earning, then he was right. I was (and still am) powerful and potent; in traditional terms, a 'phallus bearer'. As many able women do (and indeed have, throughout the centuries), I had been hiding my rebellion under a giving, modest exterior. I had been bullied through school and my early working life in a way that I believe no male would have been for being this way. I had learned to isolate my potency in mostly solo pursuits (completing degrees, writing books, indulging in art and music in my own home). I went about the world in fear of being punished if people realised just how strong and able I was. My husband's infidelity felt like a smashing, vengeful fist to show I had not hidden my 'potential for action' well enough.

From the start, I carried the fear of revenge into the consulting room. I felt sure that at some point my analyst would find me intolerably threatening and would attack, criticising me or possibly ending the treatment. I felt safest when I was crying because I thought he would feel more comfortable if he believed he was stronger than me. I instinctively tried to protect myself: scanning for signs of rage or disquiet and making sure he knew I respected

DOI: 10.4324/9781003326700-4

him professionally and intellectually (genuine respect, but very consciously communicated). I drip-fed tests of trust by gradually sharing evidence of my strength of character, intellect and achievements. He kept responding as if none of these things pained him. He did not pounce. Feeling cautiously relieved and liberated, I tiptoed onwards.

In counterpart, I became aware of my own discomfort at how powerful *he* seemed. He was an expert in a field of which I knew nothing. I had only the vaguest idea of what therapy involved and was completely unaware of psychoanalysis. From the start, he was witness to my very unfamiliar disintegration. He was able to observe feelings in me I was barely aware of, while giving absolutely nothing away about himself. He wouldn't even answer me when I asked him how he was at the start of sessions; my attempts to 'scan for danger' were foiled. I was feeling like a beaten-up animal, cowering in a corner, my normal resilience shot; I knew that any blow from him would do me in, and I kept expecting one.[1] None came.

There is much written on the asymmetric power dynamics of the dyad and their regressive effects on the patient. I felt this acutely. For me, it was not just a retreat into the debilitating vulnerability of childhood, but also into the more passive vulnerability of a classic 'receiving' womanhood, with which I was out of touch. Essentially, I felt engaged in a subtle battle for primacy. In many ways, he easily won this at the start (and I wanted him to, so that I could stay safe). But as I weathered the most eviscerating storms of grief, my strength grew, and with it my fear.

An email exchange captured the intensity and erotic nature (for me, anyway) of this quiet battle. With a regular time in the diary, there had been no need for any written correspondence since our first consultation, and it was not our habit to greet each other by name. So, it was a few months after treatment began, when I first wrote to him with a date query using his and my first names – as I would with everyone in my life. He wrote back, addressing me as 'Ms Moore', and signed with his full name.

Unfamiliar with the naming norm in the field, this sparked rich imaginings prior to my next session. I felt rejected and confused. Had I misunderstood that I was meant to share myself intimately and openly with him? Was he trying to tell me I was getting it wrong? It felt fake and anxious – almost an accusation that I was not to be trusted to respect the boundaries in the room. Or did he not trust himself? The first possibility felt insulting, the second frightening. Why did he want to address me as if he knew me no better than his bank manager? Why should I not call him by his name, when he no doubt gives his first name to the Starbuck's attendant preparing his coffee?

I also felt he had tried to put me in my place – or rather, someone *else*'s. How could he forget I had a PhD? We had discussed my academic achievements in session. Did he *want* to forget? 'Ms Moore' sounded very junior and inextricably feminised. Was that on some level more comfortable for him? Meanwhile, was I to call him Mr or Dr? At this point, I did not know whether he had a PhD/MD. I hoped he did, as I thought he would be less likely to resent my own qualifications, but the thought of being made to greet him by either title felt nothing short of sexually sadistic. For 'Mr', I had a strong image of him as an abusive schoolteacher – first encouraging me, the schoolgirl, to open up and share intimate sexual details about myself, then telling me to bend over a desk for a whipping. The thought of calling him 'Dr' made me think he wanted me on my knees in front of him in a nurse's outfit, ready to service him and pay homage. The idea of us both calling each other 'Dr' felt more tolerable, but rather ridiculous – I had an image of us battling it out across the couch with Star-Wars-style lightening rods. (I think it was later that I tripped on Gorkin's phrase "phallic jousting" (1985) to describe one dynamic that may arise when analysts deal with phallic characters.)

When I came back into session, I found myself sharing a watered-down version of these thoughts; early in the analysis and fearing my analyst's distaste, I did not feel able to share the sexual imagery at all.[2] The discussion we did have revealed fruitful resonances in the past of my parents withdrawing their affection when I'd been bad. I also remember now that I did have to call my father by his surname at times; he was a visiting teacher for my primary school class as a young child.

My analyst's presence has been overwhelmingly calm and unforceful throughout my treatment, though not without huge impact. Nevertheless, it felt that this 'phallic jousting' continued through the first 9 months – in my mind at least, if not in his. When I felt annoyed with him, I found myself wanting to talk about my business career. And one day, in a more intense flurry of angry resistance, I imagined striding into his office, pulling out my miraculously sprouted 2ft penis and challenging him to 'beat that'![3] I mentioned this explicit image only much later, just saying at the time that I was feeling a certain, fleeting competitiveness.

The image surprised me though; I had not been conscious of this potency-based aggression before, and it was in marked contrast to my actual struggle to assert myself in most of my real relationships. It felt a little like having a caged animal within me that would wreak havoc if allowed out (a stallion, dare I say it).

Gratitude was the emotion I was most comfortable feeling and expressing to my analyst at this time. It was very sincere; yet could it be an antidote to this aggression? One could speculate that gratitude is an effective way of handing over potency to my analyst – thus contributing to my sense of safety and suppressing the aggressive instincts which we women are told so clearly by society that we should not have.

Starting to read the psychoanalytic literature may have been a less direct way for me to express this aggression. I did this for many reasons, starting a few months in. In part, it simply reflected my long-established love of learning and helped me glean numerous insights into my own psychology. In part, it was a powerful coping technique – helping me accept the bewildering and frightening emotions I was feeling in the room and embrace them as allowable. It also acted as a way of maintaining psychological contact with my analyst between sessions and trying to understand better what might be in his mind. It could be seen, too, as an attempt on the daughter's part to grow up in her father's image – My father was my first piano teacher, an instrument I studied to expert level, so the 'apprenticeship' model is a natural one for me.

Another function, however, was to rebalance the power in the room and take ownership of my own journey. While it never felt consciously aggressive on my part, it could certainly be interpreted as a grab for potency – encroaching on his area of expertise and source of intellectual control, taking the 'fight for supremacy' to his home territory, while threatening to stop needing him by claiming some of the analytic function for myself.

Beginning to write could be seen as upping the ante even further, providing a rather delicious study of the interrelation between love, gratitude and aggression. In terms of love, it was a valuable way to bridge the emptiness and maintain a sense of connection through breaks. In terms of gratitude, it pays testament to all we achieved and how important and finely attuned his contribution was. Yet camouflaged, perhaps by this, was aggression: was I 'othering' him in his own field; a healing antidote to the dependency I was experiencing in the consulting room? The energy of this whole chapter – one of the first I drafted – could be viewed as something of a rebellious fireworks display, or perhaps a finely-feathered mating ritual: were we two rival male birds strutting our stuff or was I flashing my female feathers to seduce him? Certainly, there was a struggle for 'voice' and a sense that either one or the other of us needed to win. Was my reading and writing in psychoanalysis a castrating act? Or was I being repressed if I was not allowed to pursue my intellectual interests and claim understanding of myself through them? Certainly, I was asking myself at this time: is there anything like a win/win in the battle for potency between a man and a woman?

One would assume that an analysis that ends well would involve some internalisation of the analytic function, and reduction of the analyst's importance. Yet classic doctrine in the field would suggest otherwise, for women at least. In *Analysis – Terminable and Interminable* (1937), Freud expresses frustration at how hard it is to convince female patients to renounce what he calls their phallic identification. (Indeed, I am sure I would have frustrated him interminably!) Rather than internalise the penetrative, cerebral analytic function, women should permanently accept that it is not theirs. He goes on to quote Ferenczi on the ultimate goals of analysis:

> In every male patient the sign that his castration-anxiety has been mastered must be forthcoming, and this sign is a sense of equality of rights with the analyst; and every female patient, if her cure is to rank as complete and permanent, must have finally conquered her masculinity-complex and become able to submit without bitterness to thinking in terms of her feminine role.
>
> (Freud 1937, Collected Papers, S.*)

This sounds a smidgen like Freud's and Ferenczi's own wish fulfilment to me! (It is lovely being a lay patient; one can be irreverent toward even the biggest daddies of them all. . . .)

Times have certainly moved on. And it is probably too easy to take potshots at the writings of a century ago, however perceptive they were for the time. Our task must be to rigorously debate and update for our own time – just as we might add amendments to a constitution. Have we done so in full? Are we absolutely clear about the self-conception, or the relation to the male analyst that we are trying to help our female analysands achieve?

My analyst never made any attempt to constrain my reading or expressed any concern about it. When I expressed my own anxiety that he might object, he sounded puzzled and observed "it is as if you feel I would not want you to develop"? Perhaps this was an act of reparenting – consciously designed or otherwise. My anxiety may have been entirely a transference reaction based on my father's desire to maintain his authority and status over me. Or it may be based on my experience in a previous career of senior colleagues' hostility to my advancement. But certainly, I entered analysis afraid that I would be punished for being a strong, able woman; as I said to him once, "I play deferent, so people don't freak out".

How I felt about my classically masculine and feminine aspects at the beginning of therapy was reflected closely, I told him, in my attitude to playing the piano and harp. The piano allowed me uninhibited expression. It was solid and unbreakable, so I could play it as hard as I wanted, with a huge range of dynamic and musical expression. Piano repertoire was diverse and written by all the greats of the musical pantheon, so the emotional and musical satisfaction was far greater. I could throw my whole body into playing and expressing myself in an unrestrained way. But I did so relatively secretly – I rarely played in public, and I played overwhelmingly for pleasure when alone – tackling difficult pieces and enjoying the collision of my physical, emotional and intellectual selves in free, unfettered expression.

The harp, by contrast, was for me like going out wearing a dress, with heels and makeup. It was there to please others. People wanted to hear me play the harp because it was so 'beautiful', 'romantic', even 'angelic'. Yet the range of repertoire and musical expression is far more limited. Playing well is a highly restrained process. You have to pay great attention not to buzz strings against your nails. The harp rests on your shoulder so you cannot move in an unrestrained way, or it will fall off. The harp is fragile, and strings break constantly. Indeed, the instrument had sat neglected, gathering dust and with broken strings for many years in my living room. I associated the harp with how I viewed my relationship to the stereotypically feminine – inadequate, uncomfortable, constrained and ultimately neglected.

I told him if I had to choose, it was piano every time. I really didn't like harp much at all. He queried whether it needed to be one or the other, suggesting that "ors could be ands";[4] a more liberated view than Freud's.

'Ors can be ands' became one of my mantras for exploring layers of myself, including my erotic identity, throughout my therapy. It was one of many 'permissions to open'.

Notes

1 In his 1919 paper *Lines of Advance in Pyschoanalytic Therapy,* Freud discusses patients' elevated state of vulnerability and the analyst's responsibility: "It is the analyst's task not to disturb their holding or containing function (e.g. through a counter-transference enactment) otherwise the patient will experience an intolerable increase in signal anxiety and felt danger". That phrase 'signal anxiety' captures perfectly the inner, gut-driven fright patients grapple with. In my lay terms, the patient has an 'animal self', which constantly scans for danger and can take fright at even the subtlest rustle in the analyst's psychological undergrowth. I believe one of the greatest and most essential services an analyst can offer their patients is to consistently scan this 'undergrowth' for branches that may snap at the worst moment for their vulnerable patients.

2 In the analytic literature, the focus tends to be on the unconscious feelings within the patient that the analyst observes and makes conscious to the patient. There is understandably very little discussion of what the patient *doesn't* say (i.e. what is conscious for the patient, but unknown to the analyst). I hope this account, from the patient's perspective, can offer some insight in this area. I have not seen extensive discussion on the skills needed to help a patient speak, while of course maintaining the proper level of withholding, i.e. making it hard to speak but possible enough to make that breakthrough. The experience of being afraid of revealing, managing to speak and being received with calm compassion is one of the most powerful, therapeutic processes for growth – reparation against the experiences of reprisal and shame we felt for being 'fully ourselves' as children. This is the essence of 'the talking cure' – and perhaps particularly important in salving the silencing many women patients have endured through their lives.

3 In telling of my 'imagined 2ft penis', I know I am offering ample fodder for interpretations of 'penis envy', a concept much debated over the last century and

maligned by many feminist commentators. Dismissing it entirely is tempting for me, but probably pointless. ("The lady doth protest too much?") I will say, however, that the dominance and oversimplification of penis envy as a narrative can obscure other readings and nuances. For those with the appetite to examine the literature in this area, Breen's 1993 edited volume, *The Gender Conundrum*, and Saguaro's 2000 reader on *Psychoanalysis and Woman* provide useful starting points. Benjamin (1988) offers an interesting reworking around the concept of submission. Balsam (2012) provides a rich, feminist reframing of how analysts can better support women's explorations of their gender identity through female body-centric interpretations. Celenza (2014) offers a framing of gender identity which is more flexible, and feels more true to me as a patient, than Freud's or Lacan's. She explains: "The mind naturally perceives contrasts, but in reality there is a multidimensionality and seemingly endless variety within. So we must hold these polarities (of masculine and feminine) lightly, always with the knowledge that the reality is much more complex". To elucidate personally – my conscious experience was not of envying a biological organ that I did not have, but of actually *having* an inner power (perhaps more akin to Lacan's phallus), which others felt I should not have. Kaplan (1991, 182) offers another possible explanation of the '2ft penis' moment: "In a society where there are real and considerable disparities between the powers granted to men and the powers granted to women, the distinctions between male genitals and female genitals are a convenient way to symbolize all sorts of dissatisfactions, injustices and disappointments".

4 While I know from his publications that my analyst engages deeply with the theoretical literature, I have always appreciated that he used the simplest, non-technical language inside the consulting room. This helped me stay with my humanness and felt experience (particularly important for a patient like me, who might be tempted to run from vulnerability into a more reassuring intellectualism). It also reassured me he was not simply lazily waiting to stick whatever I did or said into its most convenient, cerebrally limiting box. 'Ors can be ands' is a good example of this. Some time after he said this, I found a passage by Celenza (2014, 12–14) which expresses in more theoretical terms this stance toward gender identity within psychoanalysis: "In my clinical experience, I have come to believe that everyone must reckon with . . . their capacity for *receptivity and potency*, accessibility and force, openness and backbone. Put as a more traditional stereotype: the feminine and masculine within us all. These binaries, split in two for psychic clarity only, function in dialectic relation: that is, they define and imply each other by contrast and play against each other as they mutually deepen. Various self-states can be described in terms of the degree to which the phenomenal experience is *receptive* (feelingful) and *potent* (agentic). A healthy state of mind is maximally both . . . the poles are not actually opposite (thereby are not mutually exclusive). . . . One aim of clinical practice is to liberate our patients from constraint and degradation in the construction of self-referents. . . . This expansion involves the acceptance and inclusion of binarial, oppositional categories in a 'both/and' multiplicity, in effect to achieve a *unique gender blend*". (Author's own italics.)

References

Balsam, R. (2012) *Women's Bodies in Psychoanalysis*. New York: Routledge.

Benjamin, J. (1988) *The Bonds of Love*. London: Virago Books.

Breen, D. (ed.) (1993) *The Gender Conundrum: Contemporary Psychoanalytic Perspectives on Femininity and Masculinity*. London: Routledge.

Celenza, A. (2014) *Erotic Revelations, Clinical Applications and Perverse Scenarios*. New York: Routledge.

Freud, S. (1937) 'Analysis terminable and interminable', in *Standard Edition Vol. 23*. London: Hogarth Press.

Gorkin, M. (1985) 'Varieties of sexualised Countertransference.' In *Pyschoanalytic Review*, 72(3), 421–440.

Kaplan, L. (1991) *Female Perversions*. New York: Doubleday.

Seduction

"Have you ever considered using the couch?"

Four months in, 10 minutes before the end of my session, before I took a week off to travel in Africa, my analyst looked me straight in the eyes and asked whether I had ever considered using the couch.

Three things had happened earlier in the session, which may or may not have prompted his initiative. I had expressed embarrassment and the desire not to look at him while telling him of a dream I'd had about my husband, transformed into a dwarf, trying to have sex with me. ("He was much diminished and not able to satisfy me", I'd laughed shyly.) I had then told him about my academic achievements, including a story about a fellow MBA student who had said he'd felt his balls had been cut off after failing to keep up with me when solving a maths problem (said with loneliness, above all else). (Note my stressing of 'shy' and 'lonely' so that you, the reader, don't also start to hate me). Finally, I'd come over to his side of the room for the first time to show him a photo on my iPhone of the new car I was buying – a rather dashing looking convertible. Our hands had touched fractionally on handing over the iPhone. I felt unnerved being in his space and went back to my side of the room, which also felt uncomfortable, as I had to come over again to collect my iPhone a few seconds later. I was a little like a cat on a hot tin roof.

It was then that he asked me about the couch. I had never even seen the couch. It was right there, facing me, beside him. But I hadn't noticed it. There were only three items of furniture in the sparse room, so I must have blocked it out! It felt like he'd just told me there was a bed in the room – not because he wanted to seduce me, but because he wanted to show that he could. I felt thrown back into young, inexperienced femininity. It felt like an aggressive, predatory act – a grab for the potency in the room.

Even worse, he explained that he would sit behind my head. He was allowed to be unseen, closing down the fragments of knowing him I could

DOI: 10.4324/9781003326700-5

glean from looking at him – while I was stripped bare. It felt like he was trying to teach me to submit to my man. "I am feeling very threatened", I managed to say to him. "You already have so much power".

"Mmm", he agreed.

I said categorically that no, I would never use the couch. And I was struck by just how afraid I felt.

The next day was one of the most anxious of my life. My fear scared me. How could I be healthy if I was this scared of a couch? Had something happened to me I hadn't known about to explain this fear? With my family already torn apart, was it about to be torn further? I had a fundamental fear that I wouldn't be able to escape this man – that I'd be forced to share things with him and discover things I didn't want to, that he had me cornered and wouldn't let me get away.

But I am someone who picks up gauntlets when they are thrown down. I am also a pleaser. Like a young girl not sure whether she's ready to kiss on a second date, but unable to stick to a 'no', I didn't want him to feel I was wasting his time. I didn't want him to lose patience with me. I didn't feel okay about saying 'I don't understand this' or 'I'm not ready'.

When I returned from Africa, I said I was willing to try, but I really didn't want him behind my head. He gently refused to move, and without time to think, I lay down anyway. He dimmed the lights above me so they weren't dazzling. The light at his seat stayed on. I told him I didn't know how long I could do it for, but I would give it a try. The next session, I expected to come in and talk about whether I would sit or lie down, but the room was already set up for lying down, with the lights low and the chair pushed right back. He assumed I'd lie with him again . . . so I did.

I was struck by just how much he could get me to do, with little more than a nudge.

Penetration

"You are now the man I've been second most intimate with in my life. It is a barren feeling to have with a total stranger."

For the first few sessions, I lay with one leg crossed across the other. He was particularly gentle and quiet – un-intrusive. I began to feel safe and intoxicated with the intimacy – like I was part of something I had not been before. Sexual even. There was something paradoxically powerful in the surrender of it. Lying there forced me into an unfamiliar 'receiving' mode. This was a very new thing. I came there at nighttime. It was very isolated. I began speaking more easily, more intimately. Before I knew it, my legs uncrossed. And it felt quite magical.

And then I found myself flooded with loss – a loss of exclusivity with my husband. I was lying in the dark with another man, utterly vulnerable, and sharing myself intimately. I was somewhere I never expected to be, with a person I had not exactly picked – or not for this. And he was sitting powerfully behind my head, not stripped bare at all. Invisible even. At the time, I had no awareness of the concept of 'regression'. Yet the sense of being young and powerless landed on me viscerally. "I feel 17 . . . 12 even", I told my analyst, as I curled my body up for protection. "You are now the man I've been second most intimate with in my life", I told him. "It is a barren feeling to have with a total stranger".

"Mmm", he said calmly. And I wept – with a sense of loss and disorientation, and also relief that what I was feeling was sayable: that he wouldn't explode or panic and didn't seem repulsed.

I found myself incredibly stimulated by this new level of intimacy, and I began experiencing waves of greater emotional openness – inside and outside the consulting room. This, we came to call 'the unlocking'. I was sharing more with people, feeling and expressing my emotions more, feeling hurt and love more deeply, finding more joy in connecting with others.

DOI: 10.4324/9781003326700-6

(Here I think of Ghent (1990, 108) who describes the patient's emotional surrender as transformation, bringing "a quality of liberation and expansion of the self as a corollary to the letting down of defensive barriers".) It was quite an ecstatic sense of life opening up and isolation being peeled away.

In equal measure, however, I found myself afraid of the closeness of the couch. I had ended a 21-year relationship to avoid wanting a man who didn't/wouldn't/couldn't want me back, and I dreaded the idea of ending up in the same place in therapy.

Wanting to surrender to the dizzying intensity of self-discovery, yet not to the man, I clung to my lucidity. I reminded myself that while he understood me pretty well, it was little wonder, as I told him so much . . . and his observations of my husband in the first few sessions had been equally perceptive. It was no magic between the two of us – nothing that would have come to the fore had I met him in a coffee shop. And I didn't know him, I told myself again and again.

This was one of many containment techniques I found myself using with him, which mirrored those I'd unconsciously been using throughout my life. My husband was emotionally reserved from the beginning. I'd formed intense friendships with people who were constrained within a limiting frame – married men, much older men, people living abroad, a priest even. I also deflected attention from myself by maintaining focus on the other person and their issues; my very profession involves total dedication to others' advancement and development.

I had always channelled my most passionate and sensual intensity into secondary and largely solitary forms, and this increased to a fever pitch at this time. I was writing passionate treatise, painting 2m high flamenco dancers in vivid oranges and reds and playing gargantuan romantic repertoire on the piano. Playing a particularly climactic section of a Liszt sonata to my therapist became an enduring fantasy – notably passionate, but utterly safe, as I kept him seated, his lower half frozen throughout.

Intellectualising was also an important defence, and it was at this time that I began voraciously reading the psychoanalytic literature. The very first book I opened was *Civilization and its Discontents*, where I found Freud's beautiful description of how human beings may try to avoid pain and seek safer forms of pleasure than those of actual love. In its first few pages, I had a strong sensation of finding myself, as well as finding a new field I could surrender to loving (far more easily than to my analyst, directly!). Freud (1930, 33) explains:

> Against the dreaded outer world one can defend oneself only by turning away in some other direction. . . . The task is then one of transferring the instinctual aims into such directions that they cannot be frustrated

by the outer world . . . success is greatest when a man [sic] knows how to heighten sufficiently his capacity for obtaining pleasure from mental and intellectual work . . . [and the] artist's joy in creation . . . the intensity is tempered and diffused; it does not overwhelm us physically. . . . Yet it does not secure complete protection against suffering; it gives no invulnerable armour against the arrows of fate.

Celenza (2014, 27) highlights a similar process, explaining that:

Libidinization of thought is a way of using thinking to displace a more threatening erotic engagement in intimate contexts. As in all defenses, this displacement serves to express erotic longing in a safe arena, thereby evading the vulnerability and threat of intimacy.

The verbal immediacy, physical proximity and emotional intimacy, then, of the consulting room and couch felt like an undoing of this 'turning away' – dangerous and intoxicating – like forbidden territory – a slippery slope. It was at this point that my analyst's 'invisibility' (both physically behind my head and in his classically 'blank slate' approach) began to feel truly menacing. As in life, I frequently resorted to less direct ways of connecting to soften the fearfulness – bringing in a recording of my piano playing, showing him my art, reading him my writing. All of these involved turning around to face him, as well as presenting a diluted form of my passions. Drafting this book, of course, was another example. Actual speaking was always a struggle.

I initially put these fears down to the natural push-pull of surrendering to trusting and daring to be vulnerable with someone so soon after being so deeply hurt. But I began to notice tenser internal conflicts around the very existence of his and my sexuality, as if they could not sit comfortably in the room together. These tensions seemed confused and contradictory, and initially I kept them to myself.

I feared unsettling his manhood – in one way or another inducing heat – whether rage or desire. Most sessions, I avoided wearing perfume – I liked the idea of lying there, feeling sensual, but I imagined he must have asthma and I might damage him – or he would think I was trying to seduce him – which was probably one of my worst fears.

At the same time, I made an effort with my appearance when I went there. At first this felt like insulation or armour. But over time it became a pleasing ritual, not unlike preparing for a date, which helped me hold onto my self-esteem and believe myself physically viable as a woman. I also enjoyed the ritual of taking off my shoes before lying down. I wanted him to see me looking good, but also not be unsettled – attracted cerebrally, perhaps, but not carnally. Yet I also worried if I did not acknowledge him as a man in some way, or if I threatened him intellectually, he would feel neutered and take furious revenge. If he reached over and touched me, it would also be my fault, I thought. I should contain or hide any sexualness so as not to provoke him or make him panic.[1] Not that I could provoke him anyway – nobody who knew me could surely desire me?

Essentially, his potency *and* potential impotency felt dangerous. In an intriguing reversal of a patient's classic Oedipal desire to keep their analyst 'all to themselves', I decided he was married. At this point anyway, I wanted someone else to be the recipient of his desire, as I was deeply unsettled by the thought of it. In fact, I think if I had found out he was single at this time, my anxiety would have become unmanageable. Though I thought of it often outside the room, I always 'forgot' to check whether he had a wedding ring when in the room – it was a year later that I finally dared to look, when I knew I could safely absorb either answer. At the time, there seemed little room in my imagining of him between furious impotency and rape. I assumed if I shared these confusions, he would be repulsed and insulted.

All this fear I balanced with my desire to make the most of the psychoanalytic opportunity – a unique moment in my life when I could notice these dynamics and challenge them by daring to bring my full, authentic self into the room – which at that time, felt like one of blossoming sexualness and intensifying desire; of living within, loving and rediscovering my body and womanhood, which I had never fully embraced and had been largely rejected, and therefore switched off, through the latter half of my marriage.

When I imagined talking to him about sex and this blossoming sexualness for the first time, I had a flashing image of him running from the room with his hands over his ears, crying "no! no!" I forced myself to talk about it, gratingly, the final session before the August break (when we both had a clear escape route!). Seven months into the analysis, 2 months after lying on the couch, I said the word 'sex' for the first time in the consulting room and told him how I imagined him reacting.

He did not run away. The pace and the temperature of the room did not change. And within a few moments, he repeated the same word, "sex", plainly and calmly. The words I used were neither intensified nor downgraded to euphemism. I had not lost control, nor was I 'too much' for him. By speaking, I was opening up our field of expression. By mirroring, he was securing that expansion.

My analyst was probably aware of the growing turbulence centring around sex long before I explicitly spoke of it, yet he decided not to 'make the first move'. By patiently waiting, my boundaries had remained mine. And more opening then became possible.

Note

1   While these fears of provoking were most likely based on childhood experiences (classic 'transference fears'), it is also important to acknowledge the real world women actually live in. For example, Johnson, Stockdale and Saal (1991, 463) found that men routinely misinterpreted non-sexual interaction from women as having sexual intent. Indeed, a frequent aspect of rape trials involves the defence suggesting that the woman must have been sending sexual signals through their dress, actions or even sexual history. In this context, it is understandable that women feel they must 'edit' their behaviour to remove any stimulant that could be misinterpreted – in particular, in the highly vulnerable setting of the consulting room. Yet there are far fewer accounts of this than accounts of women patients attempting to sexually entice. While I don't doubt the latter also happens, I wonder whether analysts have more appetite to notice and engage with attempts at seduction, rather than acknowledging when their patients fear them.

References

Celenza, A. (2014) *Erotic Revelations, Clinical Applications and Perverse Scenarios*. New York: Routledge.

Freud, S. (1930) 'Civilization and its discontents', in *Standard Edition Col 21*. London: Hogarth Press.

Ghent, E. (1990) 'Masochism, submission, surrender.' In *Contemporary Psychoanalysis*, 26, 108–136.

Johnson, C.B., Stockdale, M.S. and Saal, F.E. (1991) 'Persistence of men's misperceptions of friendly cues across a variety of interpersonal encounters.' In *Psychology of Women Quarterly*, 15, 463–475.

Birth

"A place of comfort and rest"

In my third ever session my analyst observed that I was "desperate for a place of comfort and rest", and I had surprised myself by crying. I had always taken full responsibility for my life, as well as the happiness of those around me. I never expected anybody to take care of me, even for a moment. After discovering the affair, I shielded my child above all, but also my parents, and even – ironically – my husband from the cataclysm that was actually happening to me. Simply surviving, protecting others and continuing to function was an overwhelming and unceasing effort. I was deeply exhausted from it. One of the most achingly desirable and intoxicating things about lying on the couch was that it was the only place where I did not need to support anybody else or 'deliver' anything. As my analyst said, I could "just be".

It took a couple of months after first lying on the couch before I was finally able to accept his invitation. A new sense of peace, safety and warmth arrived. For the first time since discovering the affair and possibly since early childhood, I felt able to rest. Lying, with him sitting calmly next to me, I felt cared for and figuratively embraced. I would arrive distressed, would 'empty the distress' into him, and would find myself warm, sleepy, peaceful and feeling safe. It was like being injected with calming, sensual wine. I even imagined climbing into his lap to breastfeed.[1] This feeling would last for days after a session and felt divinely static. The word that kept coming to mind was 'womb' – so much so that I captured it by painting a huge baby, nestling in the middle of a glorious, peach-like tangle of seeds, blood vessels and golden flesh. I brought the baby to my next session to show him. I wanted to capture how safe and warm I felt. "Well fed", he observed.

"Is this our baby – the psychological baby of these sessions?" I asked him, rhetorically, as I left with the painting under my arm.[2]

DOI: 10.4324/9781003326700-7

The peacefulness lasted a cruelly small number of weeks. With one penetrating interpretation, I had a strong feeling of being 'kicked out of the womb too early' and found myself battling on into a far harsher world.[3]

Notes

1   Wrye and Welles (1994), explore this early maternal erotic bond as "the 'body loveprinting' between mother and baby [which] forms the basis of all eroticism". They locate the earliest kindling of desire in "the primitively based hungers, impulses, and longings oriented toward the mother's voluptuous and sensually experienced body" and stress the importance of breast milk, as well as the baby's own fluids in the ministrations of this bond. Wrye and Welles are joined by Celenza (2014), Mann (1997), Balsam (2012), Orbach (2000), and Atlas (2016) in giving in-depth attention to the maternal erotic transference, which has sometimes been obscured from discussions of the erotic and merged with the general nurturing or caring offered to patients. Celenza (2014, 40) quotes a patient, Malika, who describes a very similar sensation to the one I felt: "It was a kind of love, erotic, but I didn't want to have sex with [my analyst]. I didn't need that. It was a room filled with love. A kind of floaty feeling that involved my whole body. It now energizes me for my life too".
2   David Mann (1997) describes "two deeply significant metaphors for therapy: (1) the analytic couple is seen in terms of the mother and infant dyad; (2) psychological development between this pair is the 'analytic child'. . . . The analytic couple, therapist and patient, have an analytic baby, the psychological growth of the analysand (and often of the therapist, too). The metaphor is pregnant with meaning . . . [placing] the incestuous encounter at the heart of the analytic experience". (7)
3   I sometimes wonder about that moment of the 'penetrating interpretation' – did I feel it and interpret it as such, because my system needed a 'peg' to hang my next transference reaction onto? Or was there something uncomfortable in that maternal holding, that inclined my analyst to 'shake me out of it'? Wrye and Welles (1994) describe one erotic counter-transference reaction to the early maternal transference that may resonate here: "What the patient longs for is contact with the analyst's voluptuous body or with bodily products. Both participants may face the longing for and terror engendered by the wish to be one being in the same skin. . . . A patient seeking merger may regress, thereby causing the analyst to defensively introduce the father with penetrating interpretations". Mann explains further "the apprehension of the pre-Oedipal mother is that she is engulfing, and that she threatens the therapist, patient and the child with loss of a separate identity. We cautiously approach this material for fear we may be permanently sucked in". My analyst's penetrating interpretation – piercing the temporary comfort of a more womb-like holding, felt like a repetition of an experience I had had many times – being asked to 'stand on my own two feet'/brush myself off/be independent a little before I was ready. These painful repetitions – which feel an inevitable part of the analytic process – always stretch the patient to confront past pain and grow. It feels like something of a tightrope for the analyst to walk: to attempt to eradicate them would be to coddle and therefore stunt insight and growth; yet to allow them full rein, driven by unanalysed counter-transference, is of course to risk re-injury.

References

Atlas, G. (2016) *The Enigma of Desire, Sex, Longing, and Belonging in Psychoanalysis*. New York and London: Routledge.

Balsam, R. (2012) *Women's Bodies in Psychoanalysis*. New York: Routledge.

Celenza, A. (2014) *Erotic Revelations, Clinical Applications and Perverse Scenarios*. New York: Routledge.

Mann, D. (1997) *Psychotherapy: An Erotic Relationship. Transference and Countertransference Passions*. New York: Routledge.

Orbach, S. (2000) *The Impossibility of Sex*. New York: Touchstone.

Wrye, H.K. and Welles, J.K. (1994) *The Narration of Desire: Erotic Transferences and Countertransferences*. Hillsdale, NJ: Analytic Press.

Father

"You went deeper than I wanted. I tried to get away, but you didn't let me."

He had been shaking at the door handle and the window fittings for some time. And now, father burst through with full force.

Dreams started – of a mob trying to invade my house – trying to break through the front door, pushing at the loose hinges or forcing their way through double doors that didn't quite meet in the middle. I dreamed also of going to look at new houses to buy, entering a house to view and finding myself stuck in just one room with a homeless man who cornered me and urinated in my mouth. (My analyst consults from a single, isolated office room, away from his home.) The dreams started a few weeks after the divorce became final – when even the pretence of being under the protection of another man was stripped away – when for the first time since I was 17, I was truly alone and 'takeable'.

Over-eating was a long-established habit I had never fully understood or conquered. I began a phase of eating compulsively the same week I first lay on the couch, and I put on 15lbs in the following 3 months. When I tried to imagine being thin, I had flashing images of being raped.[1] The thought of being slender while lying on the couch felt so overexposed; my mind shut down when I tried to envisage it. Existing as a woman next to him as a man, in such close proximity, felt like living within a magnetic force field – breaking the rules. The 'in between-ness' of lying there, with my analyst behind my head powerfully stimulated (and simulated) a fear I had not known I had.

I realised I had shielded myself from this 'in between-ness' my whole life. I had had only one long relationship with a man through adulthood, not so much as holding another man's hand in 2 years I'd been single. I had never flirted with a man; it was as if I had an 'on/off' switch for my sexual self, which had only been allowed on in the moments of actually having sex. The

DOI: 10.4324/9781003326700-8

rest of the time, that sexual self had been banished. I was a professional, an intellectual, a mother, a friend, a writer, a musician – any number of things, but not really in any active sense, a woman.

I discovered some photographs of myself as a teenager and young woman and was astounded that I looked attractive in them. Seeing them with fresh eyes, there was a huge dissonance between the visual reality in the photographs and how I had always seen myself – as someone who needed to apologise for 'not being right' physically: someone who could and should never aspire to be sexy or beautiful. I brought my analyst the photographs. I gave them to him to hold, which was somehow important to me. I found it extraordinarily hard to say in front of him that I thought I looked good – even though most of the images were from over a decade ago. "It seems to feel forbidden for you to be attractive", he observed. "It is as if someone would be intensely threatened and you seem to feel that whatever happens will be your fault, regardless".[2] Lying there, my entire body was prickling with the sense that I was somewhere very dangerous.

Memories I had never realised were significant began pushing their way back into my consciousness: lying awake in my childhood home, trying not to make a sound so that my father wouldn't come into my bedroom after he had drunk too much. Memories of him sitting on my bed next to me, leaning in, slurring his words – nothing worse than this – but closer than I wanted him; not feeling able to ask him to move away; having no choice but to be close and listen to him.[3] I remember not wanting to hurt his feelings or provoke him or incite him in some way – too young to be sure in what way, but certainly wanting to be alone – to have my own space – a place I could lock myself away and not have to defend myself. "You felt afraid", my analyst said – and I wanted to contradict him, but I felt my stomach tense in agreement.

The following week, I struggled with a mixture of intense fear, anger and exultation. It was a powerful unravelling. I feverishly resorted to reading the psychoanalytic literature and remember stumbling on a frightening account of a female patient disintegrating in front of her male analyst. It felt that to go further in this would be to surrender the essence of me and risk intense humiliation and collapse.[4]

The next session I pushed him away, for the first time, intense anger breaking out toward him in the room. Talking about the last session, I told him he'd taken me "deeper than I'd wanted to go and hadn't let me get away". I told him I'd felt beaten up and abandoned, and that while in the past, he'd felt like my therapist, caring about my feelings as a person, right now he felt like my analyst – penetrating me however much he wanted, regardless of how it felt for me.

After the session, I began feeling the fear we had surfaced – living it, not remembering it. I sat in a shower cubicle crying with fear, feeling like a 12-year-old kid, scared of someone coming in. I visualised a session when I ended up so scared, I curled myself up in a corner of the room, looking around for a weapon and begging him not to speak because he was 'pushing his words into me'. Tears fell down my real face as I imagined it.[5] I came back into the consulting room feeling like I'd lived it and curled myself under a blanket, shivering, feeling as if there were no air in my lungs.

He remained calm, the opposite of my real father.[6]

I began to steady, but not fully in time for the Christmas break. This was the first break I felt abandoned. I curled under my duvet, crying. I felt like a child put kindly but firmly out in the snow without a scarf, hat or explanation.

Notes

1 Orbach's study (1978) of why women eat compulsively and their fears in relinquishing that weight remains the richest exploration of these phenomena: "A very complicated fear which women almost invariably experience centres on the question of female boundaries. Being fat . . . provide[s] an impenetrable wall around herself. . . . If the fat has been a way to express her separateness and her space, without it the woman will feel quite vulnerable and defenceless . . . she imagines that if she loses the weight she will be losing a protective coating against the world. . . . A woman may worry that while thin, people will encroach on her space in an active way and penetrate her". (78).

2 When my analyst suggested that I might feel guilty if anything happened, most likely he was relying not only on his instincts within the room, but also his theoretical knowledge. Gardner (1999, 133) explains: "Children usually feel that things are their fault . . . there is a sense of guilt around the idea that something wrong and secret happened, and that if the child were part of it, then it must be their fault".

3 McDougall (1978, 56) describes the 'primal scene' as "the child's total store of unconscious knowledge and personal mythology concerning human sexual relations" and Mann (1997, 139) defines "a frame of reference not only for all sexual states of mind, but also as a central structure in the unconscious". By these definitions, the childhood memories I recount here – of discomfort, of sexual blockage and suppressed desire constituted my 'primal scene' – most specifically, the scene of my father in my bedroom at night, not doing much. However, it is interesting that literature on the primal scene concentrates on the sex lives of the parents, which the child may witness (consciously, or through more subtle implication), and from which the child is painfully excluded. This perhaps makes reasonable sense for children born to middle class families in Freud's era – where overwhelmingly, children would grow up with two married parents (however unhappy), engaging most likely in regular sex (however consensual). What of the other models of sexual activity or inactivity experienced by so many children? Most markedly, the horror of *not* being excluded, or in sexually barren environments – in which all sexual activity and even consciousness were deeply

repressed? Analysts meet patients with these profiles every day, and it seems that most theorising around the 'primal scene' serves these patients less well.

4 Khan (1972, 225) captures the essence of the fear I felt at this point: the threat of "surrender to resourceless dependence" or as Maroda (1998, 66) explains "an annihilation of the self, a loss of all necessary aggressive strivings for independence and self-definition".

5 I have been surprised by several references in the literature claiming that once-weekly sessions do not constitute true analysis and will not enable a truly deep transference, regression or experiencing of the 'infantile neurosis'. Based on my own experience, this is not the case, and going just once a week meant lengthy periods of having to cope with this regression on my own. In the end, I was able to get through it and probably my analyst understood my capacity to do so. But I'm surprised by the lack of discussion in the literature about how best to support patients or temper levels of regression when they lack the security of more frequent sessions (and indeed how to avoid 'over-penetration' or the onset of major regression just prior to breaks (when not only the patient's but also analyst's feelings may be escalated or destabilised). On very exceptional occasions (including this one), I would request an additional session, which was always granted. Yet, it always wistfully amused me to read of the traumas of weekend separations when I dealt with 6-day absences as the norm.

6 Though my conscious, more rational brain kept telling me I was actually safe in the room, my more 'animal' parts (as I called them at the time) were on high alert for everything from actual assault and abuse to more metaphorical battering. None of these happened, of course. Yet my analyst never told me "Don't worry – you are safe here". The lack of this reassurance was a major factor in escalating the transference and regression to the point of the original trauma revealing itself so clearly – and thus, finally becoming resolved. As my transference fears eased, healing came with a conviction far stronger than could have been conjured up by any reassuring platitudes from my analyst. I sometimes wonder how hard it was for him to see me struggling with such intense fear – much of it toward him – and not to reassure me, never mind repudiate the unpalatable role of potential abuser I thrust upon him. To have done so might have seemed merciful to both of us at the time, but I am quite sure would not have achieved such healing.

References

Gardner, F. (1999) 'A sense of all conditions' In *Erotic Transference and Counter Transference*. London: Routledge.

Khan, M. (1972) 'Dread of surrender to resourceless dependence in the analytic situation.' In *International Journal of PsychoAnalysis*, 53, 225–230.

Mann, D. (1997) *Psychotherapy: An Erotic Relationship. Transference and Countertransference Passions*. New York: Routledge.

Maroda, K. (1998) *Seduction, Surrender, and Transformation: Emotional Engagement in the Analytic Process*. London: The Analytic Press.

McDougall, J. (1978) *Plea for a Measure of Abnormality*. London: Free Association Books (1990).

Orbach, S. (1978) *Fat Is a Feminist Issue*. London: Arrow Books.

Mother

"Powerfully holding, without fear of suffocation or merging"

On return, the room felt different. Safer. Gentler. His tummy had always gurgled. I had always been attentive to this sound. Sometimes I found it unsettling – it came, after all, from next to his crotch and reminded me just how close his body was is. I also felt fond of it and curious about it; as the only unmediated thing I ever heard from him, it was ultimate evidence of his humanness. Now, I imagined lying my ear against his stomach to listen, just as I had laid my ear against my mother's belly while relaxing as a child.[1]

I found myself sharing with him a deeper and different sense of my body – not as object of sexual desire, but rather as sensual subject – couched in the miracle of pregnancy, birthing and mothering.[2] I spoke about the incredible inner wisdom of the female body as it grew a child, of the sensations of giving birth and becoming a fully grown woman and of the agonies, slaveries, and joys of breastfeeding. I spoke of the way my new hobby of tango dancing brought me into my body as woman and how it felt to be held. I did it dreamily – perhaps the closest to true free association I've ever managed.

The sense of heterosexual danger – of trespassing in a force field – had faded. Suddenly I could believe in his calm, his strength. Yet other discomforts came to the fore. Interestingly, we seemed to struggle to understand one another's language more (is it a leap to speculate that I was in some ways, feeling preverbal?)[3] I felt more at risk of exploding with anger at him – of some lurking malevolence in me or him. Beneath the warmth and safety, there was a dull sense of being unwanted – at risk of being cast out, and that he was better off without me. The word I used was 'repulsive'.

I spoke of Africa – my birthplace, and of the forgiving, calming warmth I had always felt there. I spoke about being torn from Africa to come and live in cold Scotland, aged two. When he asked me how I thought the 2-year-old

DOI: 10.4324/9781003326700-9

felt, I found myself weeping at the visceral loss of this all-embracing mother – at the sense of being cast out into the cold without understanding what I'd done wrong (evocative, of course, of how I'd described the Christmas break). I did not feel repulsive in Africa, I said. I wept for the feeling of my mother's arms around me. My analyst observed:

> "There is something about how Africa feels for you" "that is like a powerful holding – without fear of merging or suffocation. It is similar, in some aspect, to your feelings when you are held in tango, knowing that you are going to be released, then held again. It is so powerful for you, that 'being repulsive' is the way you avoid feeling it and therefore risking its loss".

I wept all the way home. That week I oscillated between waves of loss and elation. I felt the 'powerful holding, without merging' that he offered me in the room. It was the first time I could imagine him 'holding me in his mind' through the week – that we both actually existed and knew of each other's existence between sessions. Orbach (2000, 76) throws light on this concept, as she explains "how crucial it is for the mother to carry her baby's needs in her mind . . . the unique process by which an individual (usually the mother) can exquisitely carry in mind and heart the feelings of another/ baby, enabling the baby to feel recognised and real".

I experienced this new sense of recognition deeply. That week, I became able to imagine him physically holding me; that I was neither repulsive nor cast out. And it was the first time I imagined him making love to me. It was a soft, mutual union, free of penetration – more a loving embrace than a sexual conquest; it was a powerful holding. I did not tell him about it, though he may have known somehow; I tended to assume he knew everything on some level. I realised, then, that the benefit of facing away from him on the couch was that our eyes did not have to meet. I could not imagine looking him in the eyes for more than a few seconds without reaching out to touch his face.

A few weeks later, when I was particularly upset, I imagined him shrinking me down to matchbox size and carrying me around sleeping in the breast pocket of his shirt, in order to take care of me.

Notes

1 This was the only body part or body function of my analyst I ever fixated on, but it had lasting power for me for many months. Indeed, at one point, after I had mentioned noticing and caring about it, I imagined he had somehow stopped his stomach from gurgling. It felt like a painful withdrawal, probably completely imagined on my part. Mann (1997, 76) describes the patient's "attempt to rework

a primitive fractured narrative into an integrated view of the mother-analyst as a living whole object . . . the patient may focus on minute aspects of the analyst's person in order to reassemble these bits internally. The analyst must tolerate being cut to pieces".

2 Balsam (2012, 20): "The female capacity to become pregnant and give birth is so crucial to our biological origins and so salient in the life experience of both women and men that the functional female body needs to be as central to any useful psychoanalytic theory as the male body traditionally has been. . . . Yet, the female body, and the act of childbirth that is the physical climax of its existence, have been breathtakingly marginalized and downplayed among clinical and psychoanalytic thinkers".

3 Mann (1997, 86) describes an experience of "maternal misattunement" in his treatment of Ms F, which sounds resonant here: "This kind of [misaligned/confused] interaction would go on four or five times a session over a number of weeks. It confused and clearly frustrated us both: I felt I could not understand her, she felt misunderstood".

References

Balsam, R. (2012) *Women's Bodies in Psychoanalysis*. New York: Routledge.

Mann, D. (1997) *Psychotherapy: An Erotic Relationship. Transference and Countertransference Passions*. New York: Routledge.

Orbach, S. (2000) *The Impossibility of Sex*. New York: Touchstone.

Reparenting

"You are allowed"

Though my analyst may have sensed it far earlier, it was 3 months after first lying on the couch that I managed to properly articulate the sexual discomfort and fear I felt.

"Please don't bring down a glass wall", I said. "It won't help me". And he didn't.

I believe my parents did their honest best for my brother and me. I felt loved and was never neglected or abused. They were constantly present. My father would play with and read to me every day, helping me learn, picking me up from school and introducing me to the world. My mother was a constant source of cuddles and love as she steered me through the minutia of daily life. They sacrificed and worked very hard to provide us with everything we needed. They poured lots of energy into enriching us – through books, travel and the best possible education they could provide. They encouraged learning, integrity and self-discipline above all else. Even now, in their old age, they are there with us through our successes and our challenges. My brother and I have both led basically happy lives, with good careers, stable romantic partnerships, friendships and no great self-imposed tragedies.

Yet as all children do, we absorb 'imprints' from our parents that reflect their own wounds and struggles.

They were both very strict in different ways. My mother focussed on moral imperatives and pushed me to work extremely hard. She role modelled, a selflessness and dedication to serving others which left little room to discover and indulge in my own needs. My father vigorously suppressed my expressions of anger, rudeness or questioning of his authority.

As I reached my teens, I felt my growing womanhood was invisible or even needed to be constrained. My mother did not seem to believe in herself

DOI: 10.4324/9781003326700-10

as a woman; she had banished this side of herself long ago, so I never grew up with a model of a woman who embraced her physicality. She dressed me conservatively – right through my teens, her favourite blouse for me was a long-sleeved white blouse with a high neck. Despite not being religious, she told me sex before marriage was evil and spoke of the cataclysms of pregnancy and abortions. Having skipped a year in school, I was also younger than my classmates and was bullied and overlooked for being underdeveloped physically.

Through my teens, my father and I stayed close through mediating objects and activities. We were the two keen musicians in the family, the two who liked to go to art galleries, the two who liked literature and fine food. There was always something outside ourselves to draw the energy away from a direct contact that perhaps felt threatening. I cannot think of a single time my father ever commented on my appearance – positively or negatively. It was as if it was invisible to him, or even awkwardly repulsive in some way.[1]

In the evening he would often start drinking and became explosive and insecure. We would often quietly watch his wine glass, to see how often it was refilled, and therefore what kind of evening it might be. It was normally alright enough. Occasionally, it wasn't. He was never physically violent, but there was sometimes an aggressive energy, most often directed toward my mother and brother. Neither was he ever even close to sexually abusive, but I can now recognise that I experienced an energy, perhaps of need and frustrated desire, which felt unstable and threatening for me. Often, I felt I lost my 'predictable' father around early evening.

As an adult, my husband and I were not allowed to share a room when we visited until after we were married in our mid-20s. My husband, too, never seemed to feel I was physically 'right' or to 'see me' deeply. From all directions, my sexual and feminine self had been either invisible, failing, dirty or somehow dangerous. My refuge became my intellect, hard work and apparent selflessness, which provided me with a sense of dignity and protected me from attack or criticism.

I am not going to speculate about the counter-transference feelings my analyst had through this period of my therapy. He never gave me any indication, and I embrace the privilege of not having to know. I accepted the gift of it not being my burden. What I do know is that he stayed with me. He did not bring down the glass wall (as my father did). And in his calmness and his willingness to hear and be intensely present, he helped parts of me feel seen and allowed, which had always felt forbidden, unwanted or dangerous.

The absence of a glass wall was more than this, however. And here it becomes hard to describe, because it is not something I can pin down to any word or action. All I can do is express the result of it. Without ever seeming seductive, without ever giving the slightest indication of being attracted to me, I left sessions time and time again feeling seen, related to and therefore validated as a woman. All I can contend is that he did not 'switch me off' as a woman, or 'switch himself off' as a man. He allowed us, man and woman, to be alone in that intimate space and talk of intimate things in a way that was intensely alive and also at peace. It was unfrightened.

As a result, I learned little by little, that my sexualness was not dead or invisible. This I sorely needed after years of a sexually tepid marriage and the emotional battering of infidelity. On a deeper level, I learned that my intimate, sexually-alive presence need not be dangerously alluring or repulsive; that neither his nor my desire need be frightening. They both simply existed and were allowed.

Despite his many powerful interpretations, the finely attuned presence that he offered me through this time of huge, internal turbulence was his greatest gift to me, and the most powerful instrument for transformation.[2] What was that presence? Colourless terms like 'neutrality' and 'blank screen' don't cut it. The healing presence is delicate and meaningful. For me, it was a calmness and openness, very much a presence, rather than an absence. It was an 'in-touch-with', while not a touching. It was a caring, while not taking care *of*. It was an erotic holding and seeing which was willing to engage, but free of personal need.

Space and permission were opening up, and with that, new possibilities.

Notes

1 Samuels (1999, 143) refers to the rather neglected and "less apparent forms of abuse and deprivation" he terms as "sexual deficit", citing in particular the "failure to establish a warm, shared physical rapport with the father" and the "profound psychic pain" provoked by this.
2 As McIlwain (2013, 70) eloquently puts it, "In sustaining an intimate, honest and safe relationship between psychotherapist and client, delicate, courageous art is entailed". This presence felt almost miraculous to me, and it was absolutely core to my healing. I would imagine analysts have to have achieved their own deep work on their erotic identity to be able to extend this presence to others. Those who have not, I would speculate, are at risk of injuring their patients.

References

McIlwain, D. (2013) 'Knowing but not showing' In *Sexual Attraction in Therapy, Clinical Perspectives on Moving Beyond the Taboo: A Guide for Training and Practice*. New Jersey: Wiley Blackwell.

Samuels, A. (1999) 'From sexual misconduct to social justice', in *Erotic Transference and Countertransference*. London: Routledge.

Unleashing desire

"His erection was truly huge! I thought of you as I watched!"

My opener was catchy. "Have you ever actually seen a stallion's erection? It's truly huge"! (I gesture a 3ft gap with my hands.)

We were in the last 10 minutes of a session, and I thought my anecdote about a recent walk in the country would amuse him, as we had talked in the past about my feeling that I had a stallion inside me. I shared:

> "The stallion let out a great 'neigh' then charged across the field to one of the mares. Its penis literally grew from half a foot to 3ft in about 10 seconds, as he mounted her and had his way with her. He was just 10m away from me, in perfect profile. I got quite the view"!

I laughed throughout. My analyst, on the other hand, made his habitual "mmm" sound from behind my head (elevated by half a tone, as he sometimes does, I think, to emphasise a sense of permission). He did not laugh, which was unnerving. I paused for a second. "I thought of you while I watched", I added and laughed again. I had intended to say I thought of telling him about it as I watched, but that's not what came out. There was a moment of quiet, and I felt myself once more in the force field. I switched the topic but petered out quickly to silence again.

"You've stopped", he said. And then more quiet. It always surprised me how he knew the difference between a 'thinking and being silence' – which he would allow to continue – and the 'turning away from something difficult silence', which he would mark with this three-word observation.

I try to get back in and can't; my mind has closed. We have been here before. The time I most powerfully remember was talking about the fear I sometimes felt toward my father. He had repeatedly taken me back to what was too difficult to think about. I had ended up regressed – surrendered and

DOI: 10.4324/9781003326700-11

vulnerable. It was frightening at the time, but ultimately essential for healing, as I had relived and re-authored an emotional state that I could never otherwise have accessed. I hadn't consciously wanted to be taken back, but he had done it anyway. This lent itself to the feeling of being forced, which I had needed to confront. This time, I had a sense of wanting to let him . . . of allowing him to take me. I felt ready to have the courage to consent.

"Aren't you going to unstop me", I said. More silence.

"You are asking me to 'unstop' you"?

"Yes", I answered, not entirely sure what I was agreeing to. Several more breaths passed.

"I think in asking that, you are asking for fundamental contact with me – intimate contact".

More silence as my stomach tensed and skin began to prickle. Finally, he said:

> "I think you stopped just after your story about the stallion. That is a powerful story for you. But also one that makes you anxious – overwhelmed, even. If you think of that word – to 'unstop'. You are asking me if I would 'unstop' you – indeed, if you *can* be unstopped . . . on one level, you want to know whether you are desirable, whether I desire you. . . ."

I lay there feeling like a field mouse, frozen in exposed land, with a huge owl swooping overhead.

"And on another level, if you could actually have that unconstrained contact, you are anxious that your desire may overwhelm me – or indeed, you may be overwhelmed yourself".

It was the end of the session (thank God!). The stallion story, I realised, had been far from a joke. There was a powerful, raw sexuality and excitement in the stallion's overwhelmingly penetrative act, which I wanted to bring into the room – experience with him. I had laughed to diffuse the intensity. It reminded me of my first intimate forays with my husband/then boyfriend, when I burst out laughing instead of surrendering to the shared intensity and vulnerability of climax. I was doing it again here, like a teenager taking her first steps into sex.

I was also excited and challenged by my analyst's interpretation; it felt bold and far more proactive than the passive, holding presence I had become accustomed to when talking about sex. I could see how my stallion story had invited this, and I found myself stimulated, rather than terrified as I would have been some months before. Indeed, while I had in no way intended to be consciously coquettish, it *was* a request to engage. His response was a most artful 'neither yes nor no'. This evokes, for me, Bolognini's (1994, 82) explication (quoted in Mann 1999) that:

> Every good father should at least dance a waltz with his daughter and thereby show himself moved and honoured. . . . So that she can feel appreciated, valued and admired, enabling her to stay serenely aloft when eventually confronted with the inevitable pain of Oedipal disillusionment.

Had my analyst remained passive in the face of such an overt invitation, it would most likely have landed within me as a rejection. Instead, he seemed to be saying "I will engage with you where you are right now – and I am neither afraid nor repulsed to do so".

It was exciting. But did I want to be the mare or the stallion in this scenario? Slightly to my surprise, I decided the mare, and in fantasy I finally gave my analyst the full-blown potency to take me properly, as a man would take a woman. The gymnastics in my head were very enjoyable. Considering the sexual fear we had struggled through and how 'frozen' I had kept him in my mind in earlier stages of the therapy, I greeted this development as encouraging growth. I didn't tell him at the time, though. (I read it to him in an early form of this book, months later!) This was no doubt partly out of shyness. But also, passing this new stage-gate in my mind actually felt like a resolution of repression and complexity, rather than a new problem I had to grapple with. It was a falling away of fear: a liberation.

The thought of exploring sexual desire directly with him in the room still felt overwhelming though (as he had indicated). Tantalising too. In one part, I found myself trying to discipline it – I wanted to be told 'the rules' and verify whether any of this was useful – justify the pleasure of it. In another part of me, I found for the first time that I wanted to unsettle him; break his seemingly unbreakable calm by turning him on – allowing him to experience just how sexual I was.

I played with numerous sessions in fantasy along these lines. I imagined coming into the room and telling him the stallion story in an entirely different style, with my 'bedroom' voice – expressing directly the sexuality and the power of it. Or describing to him how incredible a female orgasm feels when it courses through my body. I imagined teasing him about the tie pin he wore once (was he worried his tie would go wild if he didn't pin it down?). At least, I think he wore a tie pin once, but sometimes I wonder if I dreamed it up entirely! I imagined turning around on the couch and actually looking at him properly, and smiling, from close up – something I instinctively felt would make him blush (though I was worried I would blush first). And I imagined challenging him on the rules. I knew I shouldn't touch him (though actually, he'd never told me that), but what about touching myself? Could I talk about sex purely for the pleasure of it – mine and his? How could he actually police the borders of my self-expression?

This was a deeply sexualised, highly alive moment in the analysis. It was the moment I was most tempted to genuinely test the frame. I never seriously thought he would allow me to break it though; I think my ultimate need was still not to have him, but to know that I was safe in desiring him – to know that my desire was not overwhelming or frightening or ugly in some way. And to know that he could restrain himself, without my needing to hide. I enjoyed speculating how he would contain me. Were analysts trained in a special form of non-rejecting, non-contact jujitsu for moments just like these?

I enjoyed practising this sexually confident persona in my mind and the fizzling atmosphere it might create. Always, though, when I came to the actual room, he felt too sedate. The calmness (or 'erotic neutrality') that had been such a huge relief in the first half of my therapy started to feel mildly oppressive . . . an anaesthetic to dull the excesses of my imaginings. When I imagined channelling all my emotional and sexual energy onto him at once, I saw him reduced to a little pile of ash. My agency seemed to steal his.

This was captured perhaps most powerfully when I read him a story I had written in earlier years. I will share it with you now, as I did with him:

∞

The beauty lay silent.

Hair, like oil, trickled sliding across silk sheets and stomach flat and pure as stone rose with soft breath – in, and out.

Though unconscious, the need and desire for stillness and rest, for nothingness and emptiness, was waiting, floating in the sheer ivory drapes and the soft air. The shadow of a cherry tree's dark tendrils lay pensive across the floor, crept over the bed, the thighs, and gently caressed the slightly-open, moist, cherry-red lips of the sleeper.

The intruder, who had battled through briar – thick and cruel – to get to the bedroom door stopped dead. The room glowed golden and the naked body in the bed was sheathed only lightly by shear, slipping sheets. Sweating and exhausted from the journey, heat rising, her gaze joined the shadow of the cherry tree across his lips, the taut curve of his shoulders and the soft silken hair of his chest.

Her breasts heaved with need, for she had been travelling for some time. She first thought to wake him, but oh, he looked so peaceful, encased in silent perfection and he enticed her onwards. Need this man-boy, smooth-skinned like a willow, lie alone and unloved?

So her body joined the shadow of the cherry tree – and she pressed her caress against lips, shoulder, and thighs. He was quiet yet plaint and still yet stirring, as she took him in her arms and filled herself with his youthful charms of wine-like, desperate burning, turning, opening and closing him piece by piece until a deeper kind of silence.

And still he slept.

As she gathered her clothes and made to leave, his face lay still expressionless. The delicate curve of lips and eyes – shining, gentle, emptiness.

This way, he'd wait as if undisturbed, until his princess found him. A woman so true, so strong and wise, that the briar would fall from round him. She would enter graceful, taut and pure and kiss his flushing check. And innocent of memory, he'd rise shameless from the sheets. She would take him to her castle and anoint him as her prince, wrap his naked skin in cloths of gold and wisps of silken mist. Yet at fleeting moments when alone, through the diamonds and the stars, a giddy dream and far-flung thoughts, would pierce with silver shard. Unsure, he'd search for certainty, but no answer to his calling. A hint of guilt enthrals his mind. His body teeters, blushing.

But for now she leaves him lying there, peaceful with his cherry tree, which shaken by their rendezvous, clings to his skin with jealousy. His alabaster cheek lies still, as pure as falling snow, marked only by a falling tear, as the woman turns to go.

∞

I had written this story as a PhD student to protest and reverse the sexist tropes embedded in traditional fairytales. The sleeping beauty legend was first transcribed in 1634 by Giambattista Basile in *Sun, Moon, and Talia*. It involves the protagonist king not finding and rescuing the sleeping princess as in the later sanitised version by Disney and the like, but rather "gathering his first fruits of love" (i.e. raping her), impregnating her with twins, then abandoning her still sleeping to return to his queen. Later, after she is awakened by the suckling of her twins and the king has thrown his jealous queen on a bonfire, the two live happily ever after. The moral presented at the end of the tale is sinister: "those whom fortune favours find good luck even in their sleep".

At the time, I thought I read my version of the story on an impulse, inspired by the writing, and my analyst received it without comment. It was only afterwards, I realised that reading it brought me as close to sharing sex with him as I could. It also provided a rather brutal metaphor for the analytic dyad. As well as reversing the gendered tropes of 'yore', it could be read as a triumphant reversal of the analyst's own penetrative role. The visiting analysand, instead, is the one in the room who is freer of responsibility and with a greater acceptable range of agency. The analyst, by contrast is imprisoned; immobilised by their rules of engagement; constantly bombarded with the analysand's projective identification, desire and aggression; and forced to hear, receive and hold the analysand's outpourings without retaliation (just as he did when I read him the story).

The story also highlighted my central dilemma; my desire still felt like it immobilised rather than augmented his manhood – it felt like a way of taking revenge or seizing back control. I either had erotic fear or a desire that felt aggressive; one of us, it seemed, always had to be predator while the other was prey. This got me grappling, in a far more sexualised manner, with the question I'd posed in the first months of my therapy: can there be a win-win in the battle for potency between a man and a twenty-first century woman?

References

Basile, G. (1634) 'Sole, Luna e Talia', in *Lo Cunti de li Cunto* (Originally Published). Available in English translation in *Talia, The Sleeping Beauty: A European Fairytale*, 2014. Somerset, UK: Blackdown Publications.

Bolognini, S. (1994) 'Transference: Erotized, erotic, loving, affectionate.' In *International Journal of Psychoanalysis*, 75, 73–86.

Mann, D. (ed.) (1999) *Erotic Transference and Counter-transference*. London: Routledge.

Female potency

"She was magnificent. It moved me deeply."

It felt like potency was still a zero-sum game. Either he had it, or I did.
And society only approved of one of those options. Looking back, I think
I had tried to overcome this problem through life by using my agency in
the service of others. A pleaser/rescuer, this allowed me to be potent while
hopefully bolstering others' success and sense of self. While this approach
worked well for students, mentees or even some other women who were
comfortable being close to power rather than actually having it, it didn't
seem to work for men I wanted to partner with. I would guess the effect on
men was suffocating and enfeebling; ultimately provoking vengeful rage. I
suspect my analyst felt just such rage at points during my therapy and overwhelmingly resisted acting it out as most men would.

But what alternative potency did I have? Something aggressive and more
competitive, it seemed. Why had I imagined striding into my analyst's office
for a penis contest when I wanted to assert my power? Because when reaching for a female metaphor, I saw . . . nothingness. I needed a potency that
was neither that of a rescuing mother nor masculine in nature, something
instead centred in sexually-alive femininity. When I tried to imagine what
this would look like, I drew a blank.

So, I went in search of it. I found initial inspiration in the first Wonder
Woman movie. I had expected a couple of hours of fun. But from the opening
scene – of the little girl wanting to be bigger and able to fight, I found myself
deeply moved, longing; sensually drawn to this character – so feminine, so
driven by values and idealism, so open to love and compassion, yet so intel-
ligent, so potent, so athletic, so strong. I surrendered – deeply – to this possibility of female potency. I set out on a quest to truly know and appreciate it
– to fill in the 'nothingness'. And in this journey, my analyst became less the
centre – by definition, he had to fade backwards to spectate. For how could
he teach me this? In the quest for female potency, he, not I, had nothing.

DOI: 10.4324/9781003326700-12

I began with books. Their covers were hard to take on public transport, as they celebrated the woman's body and sexuality so vibrantly. The messages in these books made my insides sing with a new sense of presence and wonder, of flight and possibility. At 40, I had never explored or celebrated my body's cycles, its unique balance, its fluids, its nerve endings, its deeper potential for sexual ecstasy. I began to revel, like never before, in the beauty of my breasts, the curve of chest to waist to hip, the ecstatic sensitivity of my sex, and the miraculous elasticity of my body as it bears and feeds a child.[1] (Apologies for the over-fecundity of the language, but it models what it attempts to express! I wonder, if you as a reader, are feeling stultified or inspired in response?)

All this gave me a sense of power and movement, of the potential for flight – a bursting from the body and a burgeoning of desire, fuelled by self-pleasure and self-acceptance. Bringing all this back to my analyst, sharing it with him, having him feel it, was an important step in its coming into being (though I struggled to express it with the passion and intensity I do here, no doubt in my fear that I would overwhelm him or us). For the first time, it did not feel aggressive. I wanted to believe it was a richness and power that could also allow him his power, rather than enfeeble or freeze him.

So, did I give something up to embrace this female potency? Did Freud and Ferenczi win in the end? Did I surrender my 'phallic identification' and learn 'submission'? I don't think so. I never envied the biological organ. I desired and still desire power, potency, the licence to drive forward, to sexually desire, to pursue, to achieve – and all of these, intensely. I have never felt lacking in these and will never surrender them. I consider them my birth right as a human. If I envy anything, it is the greater licence awarded men to enjoy these rights free of reprisal.

Discovering female potency was a moving *toward;* an embracing of elements of myself that were defined by their presence and power, no longer by their absence and deficiency.[2]

Regardless, a vital question remained – crucial to my future happiness. Were there ways I could learn to be potent without projecting impotency into the other? Could a man feel powerful alongside me, while I retain such potency? Until this point, I had had no sexual contact with any man throughout my therapy, so this question had only been addressed in the half-spoken drama of the consulting room.

Notes

1 Balsam (2012, 20) for me, offers the most satisfying account of the woman's body within psychoanalysis, and the engagement with the female body as core to growth and understanding. "Compelling physicality – of the sexed and biological

body-ness – that cannot . . . be ignored". She rightly laments the "over-drawn separations between body and mind that happen when theory is formed".
2 Kaplan (1991, 182) captures this idea of 're-finding' gendered parts that had been previously suppressed. "What adult women and men want is to regain access to the parts of themselves that they have learned to distrust and fear in the course of growing up [which] they had regarded as intrinsic to the little person they were – previous treasures [that] were stolen away".

References

Balsam, R. (2012) *Women's Bodies in Psychoanalysis*. New York: Routledge.
Kaplan, L. (1991) *Female Perversions*. New York: Doubleday

Lifting my foot to leap

"It is like we are rock-climbing a rainbow together – my rainbow. But as we get nearer to the gold, you take none of it. And at some point, I will leave you. I feel like I am killing something".

I have left this section almost as I wrote it at the time in my diary because it captures better the visceral sense of 'being about to leap'; the emotional leaving that every child does over and over as they grow.

I have not kissed a man other than my husband for 23 years now. And even then – at 16, that is pretty much all I did with a boy. But as I come closer to resolving my grief and as the 'unlocking and enlivening' of my analysis continues, I feel a growing receptiveness – as if we are laying down fertile soil. I have an aching realisation that perhaps I have never been fully loved by a man and, indeed, I have not existed fully as a woman, sensual and present within my own body. With my husband's and my tendencies to 'contain' our passions, I think his love was deep as a friend, but pallid as a lover. I would like to be with a man who loves to make love to me and wants to do so over and over again, who feels he has been given access to something very special and wants to receive the unconstrained desire I know I have within me. At 40, it feels like there is limited time for me to find and experience that. Yet turning toward new possibilities still feels like jumping off the edge of a cliff – the most vertiginous of slippery slopes.

And I don't trust myself. I don't trust my ability to know and protect my boundaries. I am getting better, but still struggle to know what I feel and claim the right to care for those feelings and say 'no' or control the pace of things. That is frightening because part of me is very delicate; the receiving, softer part of me that we have been nourishing through therapy, wants to hold myself sacred and feels very vulnerable. This part feels a young 16. It needs to move very slowly. This me still weeps at the thought of being with another man (as I wept at merely lying on a couch). This me wants to

DOI: 10.4324/9781003326700-13

look back on her life and know that she shared herself only with a very few people who loved her and who she loved, and who were gentle with her.

There is also a masochistic, defeatist part that wants to surrender myself to the dustbin – give up, switch off the woman in me, remain faithful to what should have been. Be pure, safe, overweight – and miserable. This is the part I am trying to fight when week after week I make an effort to look decent, to turn up and let my analyst see me.

Finally, I have an unsettling (and sometimes searingly angry) feeling that I am not independent in these choices – that they are inextricably linked to my feelings about my analyst. I have just about managed to talk to my analyst about myself in abstract sexual terms, but to present myself as an active sexual being still feels hard to imagine. The thought of discussing other men, and – most acutely – the idea of coming into session and telling him that I have been with a man, feels like a violence; an attack on the unique 'us' I have experienced. To not tell him would feel like a betrayal. As a result, I fear delaying dating or ending therapy too soon to avoid the two coinciding. This would seem to repeat my and my parents' shared deal to suppress my sexual self.

Equally, I feel vulnerable to rushing it, in some kind of rebellion or excessive bravado. As my husband continues his new relationship, I keep thinking he 'has his dick in another woman while I lie here faithful to him'. Who is the 'him'? My husband and my analyst both, I could assume. I feel cast out, undesired, effectively non-existent. Yet I have intense sexual desire. Part of me wants to grab a man (or men) to fuck – eradicate the memory of my husband and my faithfulness to him, stamp on the sense that I am being faithful to my analyst too: escape this awful feeling of being untouchable.

I know there is a lot of father/mother transference in these feelings. My sex life was always secret from my parents. They didn't want to know or see me that way, and I obliged by tucking those parts of myself away. So, I know there is a level to which I simply need him to continue 'reparenting' me – helping me to feel that I am allowed. Essentially, I need mummy and daddy's blessing to date. I need to know it does not injure him, or, at very least, that these injuries are not my burden or fault. I need to know that he is going to let me 'grow up' and will allow me, with just the right amount of sadness and reluctance, to be happy (or even unhappy) with another man. Part of his job now – as I'm sure he knows – is to release me free of guilt or shame.[1]

Analytically, one could probably argue that that is *all* it is. But for me, this feels a little like ducking below the parapet – dismissing or interpreting away what is delicate and meaningful between the two people who are actually in the room.

He has, for me, been a safe landing spot to bridge and ease the desolation of loss – a safe and celibate rebound guy. When I try to visualise this, I see a mossy stone in the middle of a pond I need to cross – the stone has been safe and firm enough for me to rest my weight a moment before leaping again. But I fear that if I rest too long, I will lose the momentum I need to reach the other side. I will find myself standing, stranded, on ground that may be solid but is eternally limited and was never meant to be my new home. And I feel sadness – a deep desire to notice the moment, to mark it with gratitude and to mourn even, as I get ready to lift my foot and leap. Because there is something very beautiful and poignant about having been offered – so generously – this safe resting place.

Note

1 The powerful moment when a patient forms connections beyond the room is another important transition point within analysis, which I've seen very little reflection on in terms of the counter-transference involved. It must take careful management from the analyst to be sure they are not attempting to 'hold on too long' – either to actual exclusivity in the patient's life or to their favoured position over other loved ones with whom the patient may feel increasingly able to reconnect. It seems likely that patients often feel guilt when forming or deepening these new connections. These feelings are no doubt transference-based but will also be provoked if their analyst has unprocessed feelings around their patient's newfound independence. One of the most common complaints among patients is a feeling that their analysts won't let go of them. In some senses, the analyst always wanting to hold on is an important reassurance for the patient that they are loveable. Lacan would also suggest it ensures the patient has truly found a desire independent of the analyst's by the time they leave (Fink 1997, 7). At the same time, important work must be done to theorise the best ways to 'let a patient go' free of shame or guilt – whether this departure is through romances or actual leaving.

Reference

Fink, B. (1997) *A Clinical introduction to Lacanian psychoanalysis: Theory and Technique.* Cambridge, MA: First Harvard University Press.

Leaving home

"I didn't expect you to be here"

I dreaded writing this section. The energy drained out of me as I contemplated it. It felt like a betrayal of the magic of all the other sections – a cold shower. Yet it must be gone through. I am not talking about the final goodbye, though that also loomed as an inevitable death still awaiting us. I am talking in the erotic sense, about being with another man. My reluctance to describe it mirrors my reluctance to talk about it in the room. How lonely it made me feel. How at risk of being abandoned.

I did it all sensibly – giving myself (and perhaps, in my imagination, him) time to prepare. The romance was developing just as I went on an August break (perhaps not coincidentally).[1] Lying on the couch in my last July session, I was acutely aware that I might never again feel this particular flavour of intimacy. I was able to articulate this to him, and we spent some silent moments together as I cried. As I went out to my car my crying intensified. I was surprised when I realised why; it was because he really wasn't going to stop me. I had been 'all his' for 18 months at this point. I had never consciously had the fantasy that we would actually end up together. But perhaps somewhere I had assumed – through a word or gesture or glance – that he would at some point show that I meant something to him beyond the neutral, benign caring of a therapist. It was not there. Or at least I was not able or willing to notice it. There was nothing to hold me back. This, of course, was exactly what needed to happen.[2]

I very rarely dream about my analyst explicitly, but the day after I was first with another man, I did. He had a long queue outside his door, and the walls to his consulting room were made of glass; I had lost my place and 'the room' had lost its intimacy, its exclusivity. When I turned up for my next session, part of me expected him not to be there. It felt impossible that I could still have him while also having another man in a different way. But of course, he *was* there, as always. I may have imagined or projected it, but

DOI: 10.4324/9781003326700-14

he felt a little distant – taken by surprise even, which was strange because we had spoken about it (was he so indifferent he had forgotten? Or is forgetting meaningful, too?). I was distant too, feeling the need to protect this new kernel of happiness and fearing he would 'analyse it away' somehow: not let me have it.

The second session afterwards, we felt more 'ourselves' again. He sometimes would lean closer to me in his chair as he spoke. I would hear his voice right at my ear, and his body would feel so close, I could almost imagine its warmth. I treasured those moments; they were especially intimate, and they reassured me that he had not withdrawn. He leant toward me in that second session for a few moments. I felt huge relief. I had not been cast out.

Despite this, I felt tongue-tied and cruel. I could not express my happiness or sexual joy. I expected him to lose all empathy for me. It felt like taunting him for the impotency imposed on him in the room. Having desire and fulfilling that desire felt brutal and unforgiveable. Yet he did forgive it. Or rather he communicated, without words, that no forgiveness was needed. He demonstrated that once again, I was allowed and that everything – or most things – remained sayable. With this, the unthinkable had become thinkable – doable even, and in the end, with surprising ease. I felt no explicit conflict, as I would have done if I had been interested in two different men in 'real life'. Never when I was with my date did I wish he were my analyst. In fact, I revelled in the realness, the reciprocity, the free flow of expression and the physical satiation that I could never access in the consulting room. I was no longer stranded. I had reached the other side of the pond.

I felt much more the viable woman.

Notes

1 There is of course extensive literature concerning patients' behaviour around breaks – including patients' seeking sexual or romantic couplings in an attempt to compensate (or retaliate) for their therapist's absence. While undoubtedly this can lead to 'acting out' and all kinds of misguided sexual indiscretions, it can also be transformative. The ultimate aim of analysis must surely be to 'go beyond' the room and patients can be showing their courage and independence in doing so. Perhaps the reluctance to acknowledge this may be due to what I've rarely seen discussed in depth – that the patient's departure from devotion is actually painful for the analyst.

2 The general consensus has been toward zero self-disclosure of the erotic counter-transference (Mann (1995, 1997; Gabbard (1995, 1996; Benjamin (1988). However, as psychoanalysis has been increasingly reframed as a two-person endeavour, involving mutuality and reciprocity, an array of dissenting voices suggest that in specific circumstances, limited self-disclosure of the erotic counter-transference can benefit the patient's treatment (Celenza 2014; Maroda 1999; Davies 1994; Hedges 2011; Marshall and Milton 2013) . Without exposure to any other

patients, I do not feel qualified to give a general opinion. For me, though, I feel quite sure that self-disclosure from my analyst at the time would have provoked intolerable anxiety and made the work I had to do near impossible. It would also have held the danger of reinforcing the wounds I was already grappling with. These were two-fold – of feeling blocked off and 'deleted' physically and of fearing a man's poorly contained sexual energy. The reparative experience I needed was precisely what the classic therapeutic restraint offered: receptive presence, without imposition. Self-disclosure would not only have robbed me of my ability to find and sense what I needed, for myself, but would have made me panic that he was not in control of himself. As someone who has spent their whole life caring for others, one of the unique experiences of therapy was not having to give myself up for the other person. Like all patients, I felt pain and frustration at his lack of self-disclosure on the day-to-day level. But overall, I see his dedication to providing the classic blank screen as an extraordinary gift, forming the bedrock of our frame and sparking my ability to embrace and believe in myself and my own journey, independent of him. As Celenza (2014, 83) beautifully expresses:

> The only lasting truths are the ones we feel, the ones that are informed by our guts, our ability to intuit, feel, and recognize as real what is already in the atmosphere between us. . . . Knowing from that level is more reliable compared to what anyone might say. After all, words hold power only as they resonate with a recognized felt inner state.

References

Benjamin, J. (1988) *The Bonds of Love*. London: Virago Books.

Celenza, A. (2014) *Erotic Revelations, Clinical Applications and Perverse Scenarios*. New York: Routledge.

Davies, J.M. (1994) 'Love in the afternoon: A relationship reconsideration of desire and dread in the countertransference.' In *Psychoanalytic Dialogues*, 4, 153–170.

Gabbard, G. (1995) 'Countertransference: The emerging common ground.' *International Journal of Psycho-Analysis*, 76, 475–485.

Gabbard, G. (1996) 'Lessons to be learned from the study of sexual boundary violations.' *American Journal of Psychotherapy*, 50, 311–322.

Hedges, L. (2011) *Sex in Psychotherapy: Sexuality, Passion, Love, and Desire in the Therapeutic Encounter*. New York: Routledge.

Mann, D. (1995) 'Transference and countertransference issues with sexually abused patients.' In *Pyschodynamic Counselling*, 1(4), 542–559.

Mann, D. (1997) *Psychotherapy: An Erotic Relationship. Transference and Countertransference Passions*. New York: Routledge.

Maroda, K. (1999) *Seduction, Surrender, and Transformation: Emotional Engagement in the Analytic Process*. London: The Analytic Press.

Marshall, A. and Milton, M. (2013) 'Therapists' disclosures of their sexual feelings to their clients', in *Sexual Attraction in Therapy, Clinical Perspectives on Moving Beyond the Taboo: A guide for training and practice*. West Sussex, UK: Wiley Blackwell.

Rage

"He hurt me"

Predictably, the first man was not the right one. There was an avid courtship, which I needed after years of rejection, then a brief period of physical satiation. This was followed by his interest tailing off fast and him struggling to perform sexually. The latter ended in him being sexually rough with me one night, leaving me slightly physically hurt and very shaken. I would not quite say I was sexually assaulted; we had not been together long enough to know what each other enjoyed, and he stopped as soon as I asked him. But I did feel that his actions were fuelled by rage (whether he knew it or not), and I was angry at myself for hesitating before telling him to stop. I ended the relationship the day after.

The first session after, I told my analyst about the break-up but not what had happened. I felt trauma grow in me over the next few days. I came to my next session shaken with a sense of shame and violation; I felt acutely vulnerable. I wrote what had happened on a piece of paper, because it was too hard to say out loud otherwise. I was glad I was facing away from him as I read it out.

He did and said very little, but he was there; calm and present with me in the stillness. The 18 months of cumulated safety that we had built up until that day meant that he was able to offer me a sense of peace and security. An experience that might have imprinted itself deeply upon me was healed in that session due to the power he had and how well he had held the frame. He was the one man in the world, at that time, who I knew I was safe with. And it was a safety not from being shut down, but from a deeper place – a knowledge that I could lie next to him without being injured; that my boundaries would remain intact.

He was offered little reward at the time. My shame, which he gently untangled and relieved me of, turned to primordial rage – at the man who was rough with me, of course, but also at all men, including him, as I

DOI: 10.4324/9781003326700-15

confronted the frightening vulnerability we women live with permanently. We can be grabbed off the street and beaten, raped or killed at any time. And as a primarily heterosexual woman, I have no choice but to trust in partners who are likely to be physically stronger and have greater aggressive drives.

My rage was at the choice some men seem to offer us – between impotence and violence. My rage was at the fragility of their potency; at the obligation I felt to pacify and dumb down, and to prop up their virility. I felt angry at not being allowed to be my full self in case men's egos collapsed. ("I bet you would be terrified to fuck me. You would shrivel up and run away . . . and I have to lie here, massaging your dick with gratitude", I wrote to my analyst in my diary.) My rage clearly originated in my childhood but I was also angry at any implication that that was *all* it was. In the midst of the "Me Too" movement, the prevalence of sexual abuse and violence toward women and children, primarily at the hands of men, was even more apparent than usual.

I allowed myself to feel this rage far more viscerally than the rage I had struggled to acknowledge during the breakdown of my marriage. It was an important step in releasing a feeling that had previously been subconscious. It was also a step toward being willing to consciously assert my boundaries – as my right. It had shocked me that it had taken me some moments before asking him to stop when he was hurting me. I realise now that I had probably 'frozen' due to the sense of threat, which nobody should feel accountable for; indeed, my numbing shock had lasted several days. But at the time, I was aware that I had not wanted to be 'difficult' or upset him. I knew I would have jumped to the defence of anybody else more quickly, and I didn't want to ever hesitate on my own behalf again. A fear I had harboured unconsciously for decades had finally been realised in real life – blessedly on a mild level. And, despite my hesitation, I had stopped it and removed the person from my life.

My weight, which had previously acted as a protective layer against excess male attention or assault, began to drop at this point. While there were numerous related dynamics we had worked through to help with the eating, this was an unexpected breakthrough. I now knew, viscerally, that I could protect myself from assault by other means (or perhaps, less optimistically, I realised that the weight could never protect me anyway).

Orbach's *Fat is a Feminist Issue* (1978, 46) still offers the most resonant frame for understanding how many women use weight and eating to cope with their struggles. She explains:

> Compulsive eating helps out in circumstances when women are frightened to show certain emotions. These are feelings such as anger, that women are afraid to show because they are considered inappropriate

for women, many of whom have been hurt when they expressed them. A preparation for a life of inequality inevitably leads to many of these turbulent and hence socially unacceptable feelings.

It was tempting not to write this chapter. Indeed, it was the very last one I decided to include. But women too often feel they cannot or should not tell these stories – either through misplaced shame or by feeling they should not make men feel uncomfortable. But there are few women alive who have not experienced some violation of their body or soul like this, and, of course, there are millions, tragically, who have experienced far, far worse. In the US alone, one fifth of women have suffered attempted or completed rape in their lifetime. Of these, over 90% were committed by somebody they know and a third were attacked before they reached 18 years old.[1] Research has also consistently shown that up to 10% of male analysts have abused a female patient, with Celenza's extensive study (2007) suggesting the figure could be even higher.

Pyschoanalysis has traditionally preferred to explore ever inward, eschewing the socio-politic realities that act upon its analysands. However, these stories need to be told, and we must all be aware of analysts' great power to either heal or further violate their patients.

Note

1 National Sexual Violence Resource Center: www.nsvrc.org/statistics

References

Celenza, A. (2007) *Sexual Boundary Violations: Therapeutic, Supervisory, and Academic Contexts*. New York: Aronson.

Orbach, S. (1978) *Fat Is a Feminist Issue*. London: Arrow Books.

Teasing!

"You think of kissing him just once, so you stay in his mind with desire, when you are not there"

My analyst made perceptive observations all the time; in ways that seemed almost miraculous to me, he found an emotion or 'inkling' within me that I was unaware of, but which felt instantly authentic and revelatory once he voiced it. He also made observations that felt important and real but were too far removed from my consciousness for me to fully grasp straight away; they would germinate a while and become important later.[1] Far less commonly – perhaps just once every 6 months or so – he made an observation that felt so left-field to have come from somewhere else entirely. When I tried to make it real for myself, it felt like trying on somebody else's clothes. These moments were unsettling, but often rich with learning. Just such a moment came a week before a Christmas break while I was talking about dating a man, and he said "you think of kissing your dates just once . . . so you stay in their mind with desire, when you are not there". I had mentioned kissing during the session, but with reference to my ex-husband. I had not talked about kissing or 'being away' from my dates at all, and I had never thought of myself as a tease. So, the interpretation deeply intrigued me. The only man I was away from any time soon was my analyst. This raised the inevitable question – does he feel I sexually tease him? And in particular around breaks?

I thought back, and it was true – I tended to bring particularly sexual content into sessions just before a break. I had always thought of this as 'taking a risk while having a clear escape route', but perhaps its function was to keep me 'in his mind with desire, when not there'.

The analytic setting is replete with desire. The analysand has the desire to be discovered and transform, balanced with the desire to protect herself and hide. This tension results in an on-going tease. I reveal and withdraw – enticing one moment, rejecting the next. I test and hang out markers,

DOI: 10.4324/9781003326700-16

struggling to express, 'half saying' or hinting at what lies beneath, then withdrawing when he sees a glimmer of it and tries to get his hands on it. I play with the promise of surrender – taking my time about it. And finally, I allow myself to be penetrated, before turning up for the next session with my guard up, as if he took me against my will. And I do all this while talking about actual sex, my desire, perhaps even my desire for him, while lying beside him. What can he see from his seat? My hair and probably my breasts. When I turn to face him, the view must be even more intimate. If he never looked *at all* this would stray from neutrality. Whether in the end my choice is to reveal or conceal, I, and most likely he, can barely be indifferent.

The analyst also teases – he is there, but not there. He is someone, but he is also many others. I can see him but not touch him. He speaks but does not reveal. He is so rigorously covered, so fully clothed, that the most demure flash of a psychological ankle can excite me. The oscillation between withholding and holding fuels both desire and disorientation; rich soil for the transference to grow and regression to set in. The analyst has a desire to transform the analysand and simply to help, but also no doubt a cacophony of other more personal needs, which can neither be surrendered or surrendered to. His wanting me – to touch me, have me, feel or satisfy his own desire for me – is taboo, even within a field that prides itself on its embrace of the forbidden.

Few of these desires, on either side, are ever satisfied and yet the promise of them keeps the analysis fully alive and moving forward. In this, the analysis is fuelled by desire; it is a flirtation with possibility. It has teasing built in.

In the first half of my analysis, the teasing was probably too dark to warrant the name. It was more the flash of a prey's frightened eyes pulling predator ghosts into chase – a fear and aggression-driven cat and mouse game.

In the latter half of the therapy, the teasing comes into its own with more of a sense of play. There is an agency, a two-way receptivity. There is the sense that I aim to affect him without harming him and that he may do the same. It is a speculation – even provocation – which involves reaching in and playing, while maintaining one's boundary. Implied within it, there is a seedling of belief that I *can* incite desire, and that our desire is safe enough to play with. To me, it feels a graduation from fear – a rebellion, even, against disfunction.

For this reason, I allowed myself to continue the tradition by reading him a new chapter of this book before I went on breaks – knowingly, I handed him a metaphorical kiss so that he remembered me while I was gone with desire. It was a mark of my progress that I could imagine he would. It was also a mark of my progress that my happiness and sense of self did not rely upon it.

Note

1 An example of this comes from very early in my treatment, when my husband
   had only just moved out and not adapted to our home being *my* space. I told my
   analyst of my annoyance when my husband had unthinkingly let himself in with
   his keys and surprised me by appearing behind me when I was lying on my living
   room couch. My analyst said "that experience of being frightened by a presence
   in a space that you thought was yours is an important one to you". I had not yet
   accessed the fears provoked by lying on the couch, nor the childhood memories
   they evoked. At the time, I felt a vague stirring in me, but largely had no idea what
   he was talking about. His perceptiveness only became clear to me several months
   later. This skill of the analyst to sense where deeper resonances lie, amid all the
   talking, is core to the patient's accessing new levels of consciousness.

Growing beyond the room

"It is like all the theory of my sessions coming into practise – delicious"

All of this, of course, was in preparation and service of real life. The additional 15lbs I gained when I lay on the couch started to come off as I moved beyond my fears, and then more after. I continued my dating with a new, fresh sense of my value and desirability – more in touch with my womanhood and with fewer defences, but also greater wisdom. My learnings from my sessions were there throughout, helping me to take leaps into intimacy and to say no at the right times (to surrender to 'the couch' only when I really wanted).

I am now four wonderful years into a relationship that is deep, real, and connecting. We are engaged to be married and I have never been happier or more fulfilled. He is open, loving and spontaneous, unrestrained in his sexual desire for me and in his wanting to take care of me. This man would never have made it through the door if I were 'the old me'. He would have terrified me too much. And for that matter, he would not have been so deeply drawn to 'the old me', either.

If I had not learned to lie on the couch, to talk about and feel my sexual self, a few inches from my analyst's body and aliveness, I would not have been able to welcome and return this man's sexual desire. If I had not learned to surrender, utterly vulnerable – daring to entrust myself to my analyst's 'holding' – I would not have been able to let this new man take care of me in ways he and I both need.

While this book has focussed on the erotic, the work itself and my gains had many other strands. I learned how to recognise, feel, express and release my feelings. I learned that my emotions mattered and deserved attention and compassion. I learned that I was worthy of love, without needing to 'deliver' anything; I learned that it was ok to rest. I felt more deserving of, and therefore became more able to receive, love and joy from others, which strengthened many of my relationships and helped me extend a far richer 'holding' presence for my growing child. I have less fear, anxiety and shame. I laugh and dance more often. My

DOI: 10.4324/9781003326700-17

'resting state' has changed; when sitting in the garden, with nothing to do, I feel an inner peace and contentment.

These are big achievements, but progress actually comes in hundreds of small steps of 'unlocking' beyond the room: writing a new thought in a diary; making eye contact with somebody on a train; buying a terracotta-coloured cushion for my living room; sharing a feeling with a loved one; having the courage to walk into my first ever tango class and then Milonga; starting to lose weight and thinking this in itself was life-changing; putting some weight back on and realising that I could be whoever I wanted to be, regardless; letting my child jump in a puddle and answering their joyous call to take my shoes off and jump in too; starting to think that I could wear colours other than black; beginning to take pleasure in the feel of a blouse or the scent of a perfume; daring to be 'seen' on online dating platforms; saying 'no' to dates I did not want, and saying 'yes' to those I did; holding my first ever birthday party for my own pleasure at the age of 40; feeling the panic or the inner critic at each of these steps and feeling my analyst's (and increasingly my own) acceptance and welcome of the 'new me' salve my anxieties before leaping once again.

My analysis continued for a further 3 years, moving on from a focus on the erotic to grapple with guilt, purpose and meaning. The most visceral pull of the erotic transference subsided in these later years. Yet stirrings of it always remained present, imbued with memory and experience; our two bodies living and breathing, in one intimate room – together.

Part 2

Reflections

Women's power
Suffering, gratitude, turn-on

Throughout the first half of my therapy, I feared reprisal from my analyst for being a strong and able woman. I had never been so acutely aware of my deeply programmed instinct to tiptoe around a man's ego, to avoid him feeling threatened. This isn't just me, of course. The tradition of silencing women and the punishing of women who refuse to be cowed has such a long history it is difficult to know who to cite or whether citation is even necessary. (For those who do want to pursue it, Mary Beard's *Women & Power* (2017) provides an excellent starting point.)

For now, we can simply acknowledge that women's battle to assert themselves and have the right to a voice runs throughout history. It is embedded in centuries of women being burned at the stake or drowned as witches – (literally accused of having powers they should not have). It is experienced by women who are beaten by their male partners for being overly assertive or speaking out of turn. It is experienced by girls who are shot for trying to go to school and women who are stoned for showing an ankle that is so powerful men cannot cope with it. We see it when online women commentators are routinely threatened with murder and rape for taking a strong stance on a topic. Less sensationally but more insidiously, it is in the schoolgirl told she is bossy for trying to lead a game or chided as a 'know-it-all' when she answers a question correctly. It is in the woman professional who is dismissed as angry or mean when she says things straight (indeed, I've read and edited this paragraph many times to try to make sure I don't sound angry)!

It is impossible to leave these legacies at the door of the consulting room. As Lerner (1994, 118) observes:

> Cultural pressures to play dumb, let the man win, or pretend he's boss are all crude, if not comic, expressions of a more subtle but powerful cultural injunction that states that in intimate male-female dyads, the man should be (or at least should feel like) the more capable, successful,

DOI: 10.4324/9781003326700-19

and dominant partner. . . . Indeed, women who dare to compete openly with men on issues of competence and power may be labelled castrating or unfeminine and have their very attractiveness and love of humankind brought into question.

Celenza (2014, 17–18) quotes her patient, Becky, a successful businesswoman, in speaking of this dilemma:

> It's lonely being successful. . . . My challenge is to embrace power without feeling narcissistic . . . or castrating . . . or like a thief, taking success away from somebody else.

Indeed, I would suggest that for many women, the primary challenge is having an inner power that they are punished for having, not envying a power they lack.

So how are these dilemmas negotiated in the consulting room and what are the implications for erotic transference and counter-transference? I have described this dynamic from my point of view in the main story; that I felt crying and expressing gratitude would keep me safer in the earliest months of my therapy. This was not based on anything from my analyst – he never responded to either behaviour in a way that could encourage it. It was based on an instinctive knowledge of what it means to be female – that by crying and expressing gratitude, I was more likely to provoke the 'gentle carer'/ lover form of masculine attention and stay safe from competitive attack and punishment, from which I was already reeling.

I can only speculate about the male analyst's counter-transference when women display these submissive roles. There are some useful steers, however, in the sparse literature. Though quite old, the research findings of Pope, Keith-Spiegel and Tabachnick (1986) likely still stand; they reinforce that therapists may find fragility and helplessness sexually arousing. In a survey of hundreds of psychotherapists, respondents ranked the reasons they felt sexual attraction to patients. "Vulnerabilities (needy, childlike, sensitive, fragile)" ranked high, coming fourth, only after physical attractiveness, general positive traits and explicitly sexual elements. Being "successful" had a third of those votes, coming in eighth place. This score worsens further if you isolate the responses from male therapists. Over 10% of women therapists chose 'successful' as a characteristic that attracted them, while less than 2% of men did (just six out of 339). "Independence" scored even lower for its attractiveness, at eleventh.

The appeal of vulnerability is reinforced by Tansey (1994) and Field (2007), who both suggest that male analysts have a tendency to be sexually turned on when their female patients cry. In a rare and courageous piece, Field (516–517) recognises a dark undertone to this dynamic, suggesting:

> [It is] a capitulation . . . an act of submission. Arousal in the therapist denotes male triumph since the feelings are accompanied by a sense of mastery and conquest. The whole interaction is suffused with sado-masochistic excitement.

In simple terms, the analyst is turned on by being the conqueror, then by dangling the possibility of becoming the rescuing hero. Springer (2006, 83) considers this dynamic in the case of boundary violation, explaining that "at the therapeutic level, the analyst plays the sadistic role while the female patient plays the masochistic role. A destructive relationship is established between them both, characterised by the gratuitous behaviour of the analyst and addictive feelings of being at his mercy on the part of the patient".

In this vein, Celenza and Gabbard (2003) have a disturbing insight: that in over 50% of sexual boundary transgressions where the analyst is male and the analysand female, the female patient was actively suicidal at the time of the seduction. Celenza (2007, 11) also cites "long-standing narcissistic vulnerability" and "grandiose (covert) rescue fantasies" as frequent factors affecting transgressors' psychological make up. These insights stand in contrast to claims in other papers, for example the seminal Searles (1959), that analysts' sexual and romantic attraction to their patients tends to grow as the patient becomes more healthy and fully realised. Is the analyst turned on by the woman's misery and powerlessness in these moments, or is the analyst driven to escape the powerlessness they feel by becoming the rescuing hero, however temporarily? Either way, power and potency are certainly pivotal.

Gratitude has received equally scant critical attention – particularly for its erotic elements. This is perhaps because gratitude is so pleasant for analysts to receive, that there is little motivation to look deeper. However, if we think in terms of power and potency, women expressing gratitude to their male analyst is surely one way for women to hand potency to their analysts in an attempt to protect themselves from competitive attack.

Field cites gratitude as the second major instance, outside explicit sexual discussion, that tends to turn on male analysts. Unlike with suffering, Field gives this phenomenon an unexpectedly 'free pass' – not explaining how it passes into the erotic and claiming it has a "more wholesome quality". I would suggest this needs more careful thought. Expressing gratitude could be viewed in a very similar way to crying: crying is a woman saying "I am suffering – I need you to rescue me"; while gratitude is saying "I was suffering and you have rescued me". The sadistic "I may have caused your suffering, and I might not rescue you" on the part of the analyst is absent, but the emboldening of the analyst's potency is certainly there, as is the placing of the patient in the submissive position (after all, she would have no need to be grateful if she had rescued herself). I have no idea whether it took conscious care on his part or not, but my analyst never rewarded or encouraged me in any way for my gratitude. It was received with the same neutral acceptance as everything else, which allowed me not only to feel it but to question its function. Are all as careful?

The link between female suffering, female helplessness and male turn-on is clear when we look in society. It can be seen in the prevalence of sexual violence and coercion in porn through to the cliché of so many romantic films in which the man finally kisses the woman in the moments of comforting her after she tearfully breaks down or is rescued from an anguished, helpless state. It is embedded in the fairy tales we teach our children in which the princess wins the heart of her prince by suffering and allowing him to rescue her. In the cases of Sleeping Beauty and Snow White, they win their beaus' hearts while paralysed in sleep, only awakened to consciousness by the kiss of their princes. In the 'Princess and the Pea', the princess proves herself worthy of the prince by being incapable of rest due to a deeply submerged disturbance (the pea). The equivalencies with the female patient, often lying on a couch, suffering and unable to help herself, being brought to a more fully conscious state by her brilliant analyst are hard to escape.

In summary, I believe female suffering and gratitude serve specific erotic purposes for both members of the dyad, making intense counter-transference reactions likely. There is a danger that a women patient's performance of helplessness is as satiating to the analytic dyad's erotic coupling as it can be to any romantic partnership. While the ability to trust and be vulnerable is indeed a necessary step toward growth, the performance of helplessness is the opposite of what it takes for any patient to genuinely heal.

Considering the vulnerability of any patient in analysis, and the almost orchestrated levels of submissiveness and surrender that are encouraged within the consulting room in the interests of growth, deep exploration seems warranted around the erotic counter-transference analysts may feel as part of this 'play'. Currently, there is surprisingly little.

It will be hard to put this right if analysts are unable to discuss their erotic arousal toward patients. The history in psychoanalysis does not help us here, with the erotic counter-transference universally condemned and dismissed as psychopathology throughout most of last century. Searle's courageous 1959 paper led the way in attempting to acknowledge erotic counter-transference as a natural, even useful, part of the analytic process. He stood alone for many years before being followed by Davies (1994) and Tansey (1994), the first provoking shocked reactions to her own disclosure of erotic counter-transference, the latter claiming that "our profession remains paralysed by phobic dread of counter-transference that is sexual or desirous". Since then, there have been far more discussions of the counter-transference in the literature, some of them courageously personal (Mann 1997; Orbach 2000, etc.). I am sure these have done much to open dialogue. Nevertheless, McIlwain (2013, 73) cites interviews with practitioners who consistently admit they would feel ashamed to tell their supervisors if they were feeling sexual desire for a client, though would approach their supervisor unhesitatingly if the desire was their client's.

My impression is that these topics still feel dangerous for many analysts to reflect upon deeply and, crucially, to seek supervision for. To fully explore and protect ourselves from the powerful complexities of the erotic counter-transference, these taboos must be broken.

References

Beard, M. (2017) *Women & Power: A Manifesto*. London: Profile Books

Celenza, A. (2007) *Sexual Boundary Violations: Therapeutic, Supervisory, and Academic Contexts*. New York: Aronson.

Celenza, A. (2014) *Erotic Revelations, Clinical Applications and Perverse Scenarios*. New York: Routledge.

Celenza, A. and Gabbard, G.O. (2003) 'Analysts who commit sexual boundary violations: A lost cause?' In *Journal of the American Pscyhoanalytic Association*, 51(2), 617–636.

Davies, J.M. (1994) 'Love in the afternoon: A relationship reconsideration of desire and dread in the countertransference.' In *Psychoanalytic Dialogues*, 4, 153–170.

Field, N. (2007) 'Listening with the body: An exploration in the countertransference.' In *British Journal of Psychotherapy*, 5(4), 512–522.

Lerner, H. (1994) *Women in Therapy*. New York: HarperPerennial.

Mann, D. (1997) *Psychotherapy: An Erotic Relationship. Transference and Countertransference Passions*. New York: Routledge.

McIlwain, D. (2013) 'Knowing but not showing', in *Sexual Attraction in Therapy, Clinical Perspectives on Moving Beyond the Taboo: A Guide for Training and Practice*. New Jersey: Wiley Blackwell.

Orbach, S. (2000) *The Impossibility of Sex*. New York: Touchstone.

Pope, K., Keith-Spiegel, P. and Tabachnick, B. (1986) 'Sexual attraction to clients: The human therapist and the (sometimes) inhuman training systems.' In *American Psychologist*, 41, 147–158.

Searles, H.F. (1959) 'Oedipal love in the countertransference.' In *International Journal of Psychoanalysis*, 40, 180–190.

Springer, A. (2006). 'Paying homage to the power of love', in *Gender, Countertransference and the Erotic Transference: Perspectives from Analytical Psychology and Psychoanalysis*. London and New York: Routledge.

Tansey, M.J. (1994) 'Sexual attraction and phobic dread in the countertransference.' *Psychoanalytic Dialogues*, 4, 139–152.

Erotic transference

Fear and desire; resistance or transformation?

In the first half of my therapy, I experienced the majority of the erotic transference as unpleasant and fear-based; I feared the dependency and humiliation of 'wanting him', I struggled to imagine he (or any man) would ever
want me, and I feared the imagined threat of his violating me. Yet the majority of references in the literature to the erotic transference focus on a seemingly unrestrained and forceful female desire and adulation. Freud set the
tone for this in his foundational note, *Observations on Transference Love
(1915)*, describing the core scenario of a woman patient who "suddenly loses
all understanding of the treatment and all interest in it, and will not speak
or hear about anything but her love, which she demands to have returned".
This is a type of transference I never came close to succumbing to during
my analysis, despite it being richly imbued with the erotic from the start.

The skew toward the desire-based erotic transference is particularly
notable in accounts by male analysts about female patients. The writings
by women analysts tend to be more varied (Orbach 2000; Celenza 2014;
Schaverian 2006). The challenges the male analyst may have in experiencing
(or even being aware of) a patient's erotic fear seem almost erased from the
literature. Kumin (1985) stands out in talking about 'erotic horror' and rec-
ognising that the erotic is often experienced by patients as a highly unpleasant transference. This is certainly how I experienced it. Yet as others do, he
frames this as resistance.

In this, he remains aligned with Freud (1915, 167), who insists that the
"part played by resistance . . . is unquestionable and very considerable".
Although Freud does recognise the potential for growth if one can analyse the transference, he frames this as only possible if the symptoms of
the transference are overcome and the patient is persuaded to comply with
the analysis, rather than the transference being a gateway to insight in and
of itself. Freud's paper is important because he clearly denounces analysts
becoming involved with their patients and encourages an unfailingly analytic lens to be brought to any feelings between the dyad. It tends to be

DOI: 10.4324/9781003326700-20

a compulsory reference to kick off any discussion on erotic transference. I would argue, though, it would be better to treat it as a springboard for exploration, rather than a framing. I believe his work has skewed subsequent discussions to concentrate too heavily on the elements of resistance, framing the erotic transference as a problem needing to be solved. This is despite the valiant attempts of some analysts in recent years – most notably David Mann (1997, 1999, 2011) – in championing its growth potential.

Resistance feels a problematic concept, particularly in the context of the erotic. It inevitably suggests that the patient's desire for safety needs to be overcome. It puts analyst and analysand in conflict with one another – with competing agendas. It is also hard to escape the erotic implications of male analysts persistently trying to penetrate their female analysands by 'overcoming their resistance'.[1]

Throughout this story, I have used the phrases 'desire' and 'fear-based' erotic transference to avoid the more confusing framing around resistance and growth. These confusions are compounded at times with the terms 'positive' and 'negative' erotic transference (hard to think of these as non-judgement terms). In some instances in the literature these terms seem to be aligned with my own: i.e. a patient with a 'negative' erotic transference will consciously experience their feelings toward the analyst as unpleasant (I am scared of him raping me/I am repulsed by him physically); while a patient feeling desire (I want him; I am in love with him) would be personified as 'positive'. This definition, however often, seems to become muddled with whether the transference is judged a vehicle for resistance (and therefore negative in the perception of the analyst) or one that drives transformation and growth.

The precision with language is important, because I suspect the two concepts are, if anything, counter-indicative. I believe that fully engaging with unpleasant or fear-based erotic transference is more likely to spark growth than indulging too long in the 'dizzy love' stuff. This was certainly true of my own experience. After all, in life, discomfort and disruption spark transformation far more effectively than contentment does. One can't help but think of the insight from Orson Welles' 'The Third Man'; five centuries of peace in Switzerland produced no more than the cuckoo clock, while three decades of war and terror under the Borgias in Italy saw the flourishing of Leonardo da Vinci, Michaelangelo and the Renaissance. (Apparently, Welles was informed later that even the cuckoo clock did not come from Switzerland, but rather Bavaria!)

The erotic transference, then, all too often dismissed as resistance, might rather be viewed as highly fertile ground for growth. This growth can either be sparked by exploring the subtle meanings underlying a desire-based transference or by struggling to understand and ease a more fear-based transference. For me, the experience of unpleasant transference was absolutely essential in identifying my difficulties, seeing them clearly, accessing their trauma and then overcoming them. It was the very gateway to transformation, not the blocker. The desire-based transference that followed was a relative footnote to confirm and fine-tune the healing that had already been achieved. Understanding the nature of the fear provided a highway to the trauma and, therefore, to growth. The experiencing of the fear within safety *was* the healing. The arrival at a relatively fearless place (of desire) was simply the resolution – it was the confirmation that things had basically become 'okay'. Yet I can't help wondering whether the typical analyst's case study might have focussed primarily on the latter – perhaps beginning with my mention of the stallion's erection!

Fear and desire are of course related, coexisting even. My fear was undoubtedly underpinned by excitement and longing from the start, and my desire was never without restraint or fear; like two faces of the same coin, one is simply turned upward to the consciousness and influences a greater proportion of one's experience at any time. The two questions are: which side of the coin do we prefer to 'see' in the analytic setting?; and are we fully trained to cope with both?

Note

1 Wheelis (1987, 158–159), a fictionalised anonymous account, offers sobering insight into one way in which abusing male analysts may view this battle. "Violation is part of my desire, the dark underside. Might be better not to know. But I do know. The garden must be secret, guarded, mysterious. Access must be hidden or difficult or denied. I seek to enter where, though I be desired, I'm not altogether welcome. Resistance must be overcome". Springer (2006) offers an extensive and rich interpretation of this text and other accounts of abusing male analysts.

References

Celenza, A. (2014) *Erotic Revelations, Clinical Applications and Perverse Scenarios*. New York: Routledge.

Freud, S. (1915) 'Observations on transference love', in *Standard Edition Vol. 12*. London: Hogarth Press.

Kumin, I. (1985) 'Erotic horror: Desire and resistance in the psychoanalytic setting.' In *International Journal of Pscyhoanalytic Psychotherapy*, 11, 3–20.

Mann, D. (1997) *Psychotherapy: An Erotic Relationship. Transference and counter-transference passions*. New York: Routledge.

Mann, D. (ed.) (1999) *Erotic Transference and Counter-Transference*. London: Routledge.

Mann, D. (ed.) (2011) *Love and Hate, Psychoanalytic Perspectives*. New York: Routledge.

Orbach, S. (2000) *The Impossibility of Sex*. New York: Touchstone.

Schaverian, J. (ed.) (2006). *Gender, Countertransference and the Erotic Transference: Perspectives from Analytical Psychology and Psychoanalysis*. London and New York: Routledge.

Springer, A. (2006). 'Paying homage to the power of love', in *Gender, Countertransference and the Erotic Transference: Perspectives from Analytical Psychology and Psychoanalysis*. London and New York: Routledge.

Working with sexual abuse survivors

Nowhere is it more essential to be finely attuned to the issues covered in the first two reflections than when treating patients who have experienced sexual abuse, assault or rape.

While I would not consider myself an abuse survivor, clearly I experienced an insecurity of sexual boundaries during childhood. As a result, several aspects of the erotic transference I experienced are similar to those experienced by abuse victims. Dorey (1986), for example, describes the victim experiencing themselves both as the dominator and the dominated; I had found myself puzzling why "one of us had to be predator and the other prey". Gardner (1999) describes the battle against the sense of powerlessness as a hallmark of the transference experience of abuse victims. She highlights the 'sexualisation of dependent behaviours' and the struggle to 'surrender to intimacy' as other hallmarks; I frequently felt sexually vulnerable and at risk of humiliation as I surrendered to new levels of openness.

Celenza (2014, 52) also describes cases in which the "erotic longings can become defensively aggressivised". She situates this specifically in the male patient-female analyst dyad, citing the male patient's fears of the asymmetric power distribution. I would suggest that these fears need not only be experienced by men. While their nature may be somewhat different, women have very real reasons to fear male sexual power, whether they are actual abuse victims or not. One obvious 'salve' to our frightening vulnerability is to transform our erotic feelings into more aggressive forms as a means to protect ourselves and compete (for example, as I did, by co-opting a symbolically masculine form of power, such as a 2ft penis).

The act of seduction between therapist and patient is about surrender and the negotiation between fear and desire. Forrester (1990) and Maroda (1998) both highlight this mutual seduction. Maroda (1998, 27) says:

> We do not discuss the . . . need to 'psychologically seduce' the patient as part of the analytic process. As a result, we cannot discuss the inevitable

DOI: 10.4324/9781003326700-21

phases of approach and withdrawal, satisfaction and disappointment, victory and defeat, neurotic fears of rejection and grandiose visions of importance that each member of the analytic pair experiences.

While this seduction process applies to all dyads, it is likely to be more tortured for patients or analysts who have been victims of sexual abuse. Davies and Frawley (1992, 30) address this specifically.

The patient must experience herself as all: victim, abuser, and saviour and the analyst must do the same. Therapist will seduce patient and patient will seduce therapist as part of the natural process of intimate bonding. Both will think long and hard, during the course of this work together, about the nature of abuse and the differences between benign and malignant seduction.

My move to the couch was a key moment that captured this struggle in my own analysis. In the words of Celenza (2007, 44) "in psychoanalysis, a couch is never just a couch", and as Gardner (1999) suggests, this push to surrender my independence and accept the vulnerability of the couch felt highly sexualised to me. I felt real terror, completely unexpectedly. And I would not be surprised if it was unexpected for my analyst also. I had no history of sexual abuse, nor conscious fears that I had recounted to him. My reaction to lying on the couch taught me a huge amount and triggered revelation and ultimately led to healing. However, it pulled me to the edge of unmanageable anxiety and, without the highly delicate handling I received, it could have repeated the past trauma experience I needed to heal from.

It is a huge leap to invite a woman to give up her power, to lie down unable to see the man she is in a room with – with whom she is already likely to associate transference fears. Early in the analysis, she will also be unpractised at identifying or expressing those transference experiences clearly. In addition to transference fears, there is the tragic, daily reality that women are regularly sexually assaulted in and outside the consulting room by those they have dared to trust.

When we consider how many women have experienced sexual abuse, harassment or boundary violations and/or who struggle to say no or assert their boundaries and needs –especially with men in power over them (surely an even higher percentage who come to therapy) – it is a weighty responsibility for analysts to handle carefully. Yet the moment of moving to the couch seems to have received relatively little attention in the literature.

It is a familiar move for most analysts, but does this mean it is less questioned than it should be? It strikes me as highly likely to be driven by and provoking deep transference or counter-transference emotions. It also occurs to me that there is a certain ethos in the field that dismisses those early therapy stages before the patient lies on the couch as 'not real analysis'. Getting a patient on the couch could in some instances be a tempting 'victory', seized too quickly by an analyst who has remaining work to do.

Davies and Frawley (1992) offer a passionate history of the neglect of the realities of childhood abuse in the psychoanalytic literature since Freud's abandonment of the seduction theory. They call for more in-depth discussion and skill building to prepare analysts for the powerful erotic transference and counter-transference effects; Fiona Gardner (1999) and David Mann (1995) have both made valuable contributions. However, these texts are coming up on 30 years old, and I'm not sure we have yet answered this important call in full.

References

Celenza, A. (2007) *Sexual Boundary Violations: Therapeutic, Supervisory, and Academic Contexts*. New York: Aronson.

Celenza, A. (2014) *Erotic Revelations, Clinical Applications and Perverse Scenarios*. New York: Routledge.

Davies, J.M. and Frawley, M.G. (1992) 'Dissociative processes and transference-countertransference paradigms in the psychoanalytically-orientated treatment of adult survivors of childhood sexual abuse.' In *Psychoanalytic Dialogues*, 2, 5–36.

Dorey, R. (1986) 'The relationship of mastery.' In *International Review of Psychoanalysis*, 13, 323.

Forrester, J. (1990) *The Seductions of Psychoanalysis*. Cambridge, UK: Cambridge University Press.

Gardner, F. (1999) 'A sense of all conditions', in *Erotic Transference and Counter Transference*. London: Routledge.

Mann, D. (1995) 'Transference and countertransference issues with sexually abused patients.' In *Pyschodynamic Counselling*, 1(4), 542–559.

Maroda, K. (1998) *Seduction, Surrender, and Transformation: Emotional Engagement in the Analytic Process*. London: The Analytic Press.

Transference love or 'real love'?

"Deeply involved, with many strands and tones"

I thought of 'the room' often.

"There is something magical about going to that room", I would write in my diary, rather than "there is something magical about being with him". The second phrase for several years felt far more dangerous to think or feel. The patient extending their sense of the analyst's person into their environment is not unusual, of course. Indeed, it has always stirred me that arriving after dark, as I did 8 months of the year, I had to pass through a locked gate (he gave me the passcode), then walk along a dark avenue guided by a sole light above the door, before coming to rest in his warm, safe, isolated space!

Sparked by Freud's own self-confessed confusion on the matter (1915), there has been significant debate as to whether transference love is distinguishable from normal love. This comes partly from an acknowledgement that a real bond forms between the two people in the room, and partly from an insistence that all love is, to some degree, transference love. I agree with both arguments (though I think the latter is overplayed at times). The distinction between the two feelings seemed very clear to me in the early stages of my therapy. However, as the real bond grew, and as I inevitably built some sense of my analyst's character, despite his elusiveness, I felt more and more that I was clutching at straws to claim there was any difference.

Indeed, the only distinction that may exist is in how the feelings are put to use. My inclination to contain relationships and my appetite for analysis helped me largely use the feelings to grow, rather than get lost in imaginings about the man.

In my optimistic moments, I saw transference love like an inoculation – a disease with the replicative agent taken out. It was the real thing, but with missing elements that stopped it from becoming embedded or inelastic. By allowing it inside me, I became better able to successfully embrace the 'real thing' later!

DOI: 10.4324/9781003326700-22

One missing element, for me, was the inability to give. He never revealed any need or seemed to take anything. As a 'giver/pleaser', who claimed never to need or take from others, it was powerful to learn just how hard it was to feel valued by someone I was not allowed to rescue.

The most vital missing element was knowledge, as I knew virtually nothing about him other than his name. This meant he could become whatever love (or hate) object I needed in the moment, resulting in a kaleidoscope of erotic roles. In the first 2 years of my therapy, I imagined him assaulting me, fucking me and making love to me. Alternatively, I imagined him frozen from the waist down, reduced to a pile of ash, shrivelled up and impotently running away in the face of my sexual desire. I also imagined him breast-feeding me, holding me safe within his body and plaiting my hair while kissing my forehead.

My imagining of him often jumped between these roles with remarkable speed, rarely resting on one for more than a few weeks at a time and sometimes flitting between two or three in one session. The analyst's willingness to remain present as each role is imposed, and also, crucially, to surrender each when it is no longer needed, was a vital part of this elasticity. One can argue that I was accessing or even stimulating different parts of his own erotic identity throughout – that they were *all* real on some level. However, the elasticity of impressions – which mirrored and served my growth – was clearly based in transference.

During the periods described in this book, I felt very vulnerable to falling from the transformational growth of 'transference love' to what I saw as the frippery agonies and ecstasies of a person-centred love. It was frightening, pure and simple, and I policed the border between these two different kinds of love quite consciously. When I felt anger rising at my therapist, I was often afraid the border was dissolving or was an illusion in the first place, and I felt humiliation lurking very close. Why humiliation? Because through most of this period, I believed that any sort of love from me would be repulsive. Or worse, I imagined it being received with a pitying pat to the head.

Despite this conscious battle to resist love, we must remember the transformative effect of living through emotions in the room, rather than simply theorising about them. This poses a serious question about the value, versus the destructive aspects, for the patient (and indeed the analyst) in experiencing their erotic/love impulses as real. My erotic transformation involved embracing my sexual self as an integral allowed part of me. It was about convincing me – through *experience in the room* – that my desire, and indeed his, need not be dangerous and could even be welcomed. It involved a series of imaginative experiments to test the interlinked nature of a man and woman's potency, helping me practice knowing who owns what. I achieved this not only through the arcing metaphors of the mind but through the relating presence of my analyst. Doing all this in the room was an essential dress rehearsal for real life.

In fact, the idea of acting is perhaps a useful metaphor. We are not simply reading the words of the play, discussing their meaning as observers while dressed in our day clothes and retaining a grip on ourselves as interpreters. We *go through it on stage*. We feel and immerse ourselves in our characters – in fact, we find the real parts of ourselves that can serve the story we need to live through. Yet in the end, there is still a distinction between 'on stage' and 'off stage'. We must retain an ability both to be in the play – deeply present and together with the others on stage – and also on the balcony, part of us looking down and seeing ourselves from elsewhere. For me and many other patients, relaxing the psychological constraints around erotic desires and embracing their realness in the room can in many ways be therapeutic. It is daring to be on the stage. The erotic *can* serve as resistance. However, resisting it can equally stunt growth.[1]

In this very difficult balancing act for the patient, the utter stability of the therapist is vital. The therapist will, of course, have their own work to do. They must extend a presence that is neither rejecting nor seductive, neither overly potent nor impotent, flexibly masculine or feminine, homosexual or heterosexual and open to everything in between these polarities. This is the erotic version of 'neutrality', which must never be mistaken for absence (absence for me, certainly, would have been devastating). As in all other areas, analysts must retain their analytic function and lucidity around their own emotions and impulses (and those projected into them) in order to deepen their understanding of the patient. They must hold the frame even if the patient fails to help or actively sets out to destroy it. This is a hell of a task. Sadly, many fail – either by banishing the erotic from their consulting rooms entirely (not only denying their patients the chance to grow in this way, but imposing or reinforcing shame) or, far worse, by surrendering to abuse. The latter, perhaps, comes after an attempt at the former; as Orbach (2000, 29) explains "if analysts cannot countenance such [erotic] feelings within themselves but suppress or deny them or separate them from conscious awareness, there is a much higher chance of inappropriate sexuality being unwittingly enacted in the therapy".

When I began my reading in psychoanalysis and learned that an analyst having consenting sexual contact with a patient was considered abusive, I initially found this baffling and patronising. I could see that such contact would be unwise (as it is in so many situations), but the idea that a patient's conscious acquiescence was not considered true adult consent seemed infantilising. It didn't appeal to the phallus bearer in me! Having now experienced psychoanalysis as a patient, I understand just how deeply the patient is incapable of true consent. In life I am about as fully empowered an adult as people get, with extremely high functioning. I am a potentially viable sexual partner for most other adults in the world. But on that man's couch, I have had the courage to be foetal or a 2-year-old, 6-year-old, 12-year-old, 16-year-old and, of course, a 38–44 year old (the last also cringingly vulnerable at times).

These selves shift and jostle in and out of the shadows, but they are all present enough to experience how my analyst treats me. To put it bluntly (and it is valuable to be blunt, I think), if he had ever tried to seduce the woman in me, it may well have been the 6-year-old who said 'yes'. He had the power to accidentally or intentionally nurture, nourish, crush, batter, fuck or fuck with all these versions of myself. Probably to participate fully and understand my experiences and fears, he needed to imagine most of these possibilities in some way. What was crucial was that in externalising to me he stuck to the first two: and he did.

Analysts need to understand the frightening depth of the power they have and that it is given to them as part of a psychological contract with the patient, never mind a moral contract with their profession, regardless of how messy, raging or desire-filled 'the room' may get. They need to understand that a patient can dream of being touched by their analyst, while also understanding that *being* touched would shatter them (whether the patient knows it or not at the time). Analysts need to understand that a patient can feel huge pain at the lack of merging (and might need to if they are to grow), while any actual merger would be existentially terrifying. Patients need to know the analyst can be calm, strong-minded and compassionate when the patient cannot be – or indeed, when they should not have to be. For it is only when cradled by the analyst's unwavering stability that the patient can surrender all anchors, jump into the rapids and begin swimming for new ground.

In this, the 'frame' – which often feels painful and frustrating, is actually a vital reassurance for both of us. It is the banks of the river into which we jump. Any rupturing of the frame robs a patient of the elasticity and safety they need to grow. I enjoyed and needed the meticulously-prepared invoices, always delivered in the same way on the same day each month, even though handing me one when I had just been curled up weeping could feel cruel – no doubt to both of us. Despite the painfulness and strangeness of it, I am also glad that he continued to call me by my surname (adjusted to include the appropriate Dr title), regardless of the intimacies I shared and the emotional storms we might be going through on any particular day. The ending of sessions on the minute and the inevitable holiday breaks may have saddened or angered me, yet seeing them adhered to unswervingly showed me I could not shake him. Throughout, these things told me that he continued to know 'where he was' and 'who he was meant to be', which is exactly what I needed him to know and who I needed him to be.

In the end, the issue is not whether the love in the room is real or not. It is that the love is so powerful, and the patient so courageously powerless, that it must be allowed into the room only with safety nets. This means that some forms of expressing love are sacrificed in order to make other forms safe enough to help us transform. In return for this sacrifice, we win the privilege of taking part in one of the most unique and deeply meaningful couplings two humans can experience. In the end, the analytic dyad is not parenting. Nor is it being lovers. Nor priest and confessor, nor teacher and student. It has strong reflections of all of these, but is uniquely, and exquisitely its own.

There is one strand to the love that is less erotic, and I think will last my whole life. That is the love that comes from having shared an intense, unique experience with someone who does not let you down – I think of soldiers serving side by side with a common sense of mission, trusting they will get each other out alive regardless of the horrors and intensities they will need to battle through. On the part of the patient, it is the love of deep, deep gratitude for the person who, however unknown in other ways, stayed intensely and safely with them as they cried and laughed and discovered themselves, as they felt anger, dread, joy and desire – as they took steps to grow.

While embroiled in the experiences described in this book, I was struggling to articulate the emotions I felt toward my analyst. I was afraid of them and also afraid of how he would feel about them. He suggested that I felt 'deeply involved'. I then added 'with various strands and tones'. And that was right. I felt such relief and gratitude being able to say that – to put those words on it – to make it significant and say it's okay for it to be significant. Neither of us used the word 'love' at the time. It would have felt desperately humiliating and exposing to me to say the words amidst the height of the transference, when still alone, desperately short of validation from outside or explicit validation from him, and knowing, of course, that he would not say anything in return.[2] Yet the word was in my mind. Not in a mawkish, fairy tale way; I never surrendered my lucidity! But all the words around – gratitude, caring, deep involvement, intimacy, trust . . . in the intense dread and dependency of the analytic setting – they are all lifelines of love. The unique poignancy of this love is deepened by the fact that I feel it for a person I know almost nothing about, whose hand I only ever shook once, who only ever called me by my surname, and who I will never know in any other way.

I am thinking of a bird that flew unfettered for some time before breaking its wing. The bird is picked up and held – gently, in two open-cupped hands. It is terrified to be held in that way. It even pecks and scratches or tries to fly away too early. Then, as it feels safe and the hands don't attack, it surrenders with aching relief. It dares to feel and want the love. Finally, the bird heals and prepares to fly away from comfort and safety. It never knew or understood the person behind the hands, but it has experienced the love of the holding – without fear of suffocation or merging. And it has loved back.

Notes

1 More recent writers, correctly I believe, have suggested that a seeming absence of the erotic transference is more likely to indicate resistance than the presence of erotic transference would. This is particularly noteworthy in the seemingly less frequent instances of erotic transference between the male patient-female analyst dyad. Several writers Celenza (2014), Chasseguet-Smirgel (1970) and Schaverian (2006) have suggested that male fear of dominant females and humiliation at their hands may well be a primary reason for erotic transferences remaining in the unconscious (or at least unexpressed) realm.
2 Bach (1994, 22) describes the "goal of analysis as opening pathways to object love". This pathway most likely includes several steps: a patient allowing themselves to feel love for their analyst; examining the nature of that love in all its elements – erotic and otherwise; for the patient to believe their love is not repulsive and can be voiced without humiliation; and perhaps in parallel to this, for the patient to believe they indeed are loveable and, by extension, that their analyst loves *them*, despite any lack of declaration. In Gerrard's words (1999, 27), "until and unless there can be felt moments of love for the patient by the therapist, the patient is not able to develop fully".

References

Bach, S. (1994) *The Language of Perversion and the Language of Love*. New York: Aronson.

Celenza, A. (2014) *Erotic Revelations, Clinical Applications and Perverse Scenarios*. New York: Routledge.

Chasseguet-Smirgel, J. (1970) *Female Sexuality: New Psychoanalytic Views*. Michigan, US: U. Michigan Press.

Freud, S. (1915) 'Observations on transference love', in *Standard Edition Vol. 12*. London: Hogarth Press.

Gerard, J. (1999) 'Love in the time of psychotherapy' In *Erotic Transference and Counter Transference*. London: Routledge.

Orbach, S. (2000) *The Impossibility of Sex*. New York: Touchstone.

Schaverian, J. (ed.) (2006). *Gender, Countertransference and the Erotic Transference: Perspectives from Analytical Psychology and Psychoanalysis*. London and New York: Routledge.

Revoicing the patient

"I feel relief . . . a joy, even, that I have *spoken*"

Writing the first draft of this book, while in treatment, was a way of capturing the eloquence I always lacked in the consulting room. It was a way of 'working through', of coping and regaining or deepening my cerebral control of powerful and bewildering emotions. It provided a focus and implicit sense of connection with my analyst through breaks (what those of a more cerebral bent might call 'object continuity'). When I passed him the first draft, it was a way to communicate with him, of connecting in a way that felt safer than stuttering through an improvised and impoverished version of these words in the room. Some of it was new to him, and it helped me turn the unspeakable into the speakable, to forge yet freer ways for me to relate to and be truthful with him.

The decision to publish such an intimate portrayal is, of course, rich material for analysis in itself. One could see it either as a violation or as an honouring of an experience still felt to be sacred – certainly by me and possibly even by my analyst (he has never said so, but part of my growth is coming to believe this could be). Sharing these experiences, for me, affirms the growth I have achieved through analysis – the new openness, the freedom from shame and fear, the permission to be and express the fullest form of myself. For me, this outing of the deeply private feels like an honouring. It satisfies a strong desire to have my voice heard, to be seen and not to be hidden. It is fuelled by the conviction that women's and patients' voices are important.

Though we enjoy the honour of having our voices heard over and over *within* the consulting room, we patients are rarely truly heard within the literature (a rare exception would be Hill 2010). We are awarded a few lines of highly selected and perhaps inaccurately remembered quotes every few pages (a little similar to the treatment I have awarded my analyst here). We are stripped of tone and all but the barest of contexts, and we are revealed the way the author wants us to be, rather than how we may want to be ourselves.

DOI: 10.4324/9781003326700-23

What we really meant, or what we *didn't* say as we lay there, struggling to speak, are only guessed at. We are interpreted (and inevitably distorted) in the mind of our analyst, and then – if we make it there – we are unnamed, merged or fictionalised in discussions and publications. It feels like a deep level of 'devoicing', and a tragic loss of insight – ironic in a profession that is so dedicated to the analysand's unfettered expression.

There seems to be a prevalent sense in the field that we patients 'know not what we say and mean'. Indeed, the very ideal of free association holds implicit the belief that any conscious analysis and presentation by the analysand will provide a barrier to the truth, rather than a gateway. The thinking, the interpretation and therefore the case studies and research papers are the analyst's job.

With a doctorate in anthropology, this evokes memories from my own field. In ethnography up to the 1970s or so, we too set out to study the 'other'. We observed, and we made interpretations about the other's history and way of being. The other was seen. We were not. The scholar's own subjectivity was not considered part of the story – their observations were assumed to be objective and correct (or if they were not, this was considered a failing – just as counter-transference was originally seen as a distortion to be suppressed rather than learned from). Most ethnographers worked alone, in isolated parts of the world, and their reports were the only source of authority. Traditionally, the other always had less power – often from 'traditional' tribes, ethnic minorities or marginalized groups. We assumed they led their lives without consciously constructing them or analysing meaning. And indeed, we preferred them to do so, so we could observe unobstructed. It was for us, with our scholarly background, to watch, listen and to use our expertise to report and selectively draw meaning from our observations.

Since then, the role of the scholar has been questioned and revised. Just as it is now the norm for analysts to discuss their counter-transference with colleagues and understand their subjectivity's inevitable effect on their patient, the modern ethnography scholar is obliged to place themselves within their texts, considering not only the ways in which their observations may be slanted, but also the way their very presence and participation will have changed what actually happened. One way in which ethnography has outstripped psychoanalysis, however, is in its attempts to integrate the 'voices of the other' in its scholarship. Co-written books, lengthy quotes – (not just overheard speech, but subjects' conscious interpretations and explanations of meaning in their lives), recordings of voices and performances, online and offline communities and conversations abound. This has blurred the line between 'the studied' and 'the studiers', with the 'studiers' far more accountable to those they represent than in previous decades.

There is no such dynamic challenge and 'cross-pollination' in psychoanalysis that I am aware of. While the relational school would now view analysis and interpretation within sessions as a co-production and recognise the illusion of authoritative truth, the analysis of analysis remains largely a monologue. Post analysis, there are two different communities. One is populated by analysts, conversing with one another through journals, books and conferences, largely describing their successes. Respect and caring for patients abound in these conversations – reading them as a patient has been hugely affirming. But as holders of knowledge and insight, we remain largely unheard. Patients' attempts to make meaning of their analyses occupy very different spaces, living in online chat forums, which are often skewed toward those who feel their analysts failed them, and lack any great psychoanalytic insight.

Psychoanalysis has specific challenges, of course, with its commitment to confidentiality and its need to maintain a safe frame for the analysand, free of pressure or exploitation – even after their treatment concludes. The delicacy and importance of what we are trying to do far exceeds what is at stake in most anthropological study. However, psychoanalysis' strict boundaries *are* blurred in the case of trainees, who join the analytic community and in many cases gradually evolve to relate to their analysts as colleagues. Indeed, of the limited in-depth accounts of analysands' experiences, most of these come from those who have become analysts themselves (e.g. Tessman 2003). While this may give their descriptions an assumed analytic authority, their analytic knowledge, the training context of their analyses and their need to represent themselves within their professional community (or indeed their sense of betrayal by that community, e.g. Masson 2012) are all reasons for conscious and unconscious distortion.

Needless to say, lay analysands also have numerous reasons not to see clearly. I have highlighted some of my own, and I may well see others in time. No doubt there are more my analyst (and indeed my readers) could add. Beyond my normal human subjectivity, I am sure that my lack of training and experience will have resulted in errors and misunderstandings in this book that few psychoanalysts would have made. Yet, this is no reason to be silenced: providing an honest snapshot of 'where one is' when one is there is all any of us can ever do. And I am confident that my perceptions as a lay patient – however distorted and imperfect – are also valuable for their difference. In the end, neither group has access to an absolute truth, if there is any such thing. It is simply that in searching to understand the richly diverse experiences of analysands and the role we each take in shaping that experience, it is vital we include the voices of normal analysands.

I believe this is doubly true when exploring the erotic transference and counter-transference. First, if only analysts are sharing their views and experiences of the male analyst-female analysand dyad, then this powerful male-female interchange is being reported exclusively by men. There are many brilliant female analysts, but their publications focus understandably much more on other configurations. Second, the potential costs of getting it wrong are very high. With a marked proportion of analysts self-reporting their abuse of patients (the highest instance within the male analyst-female patient dyad), there is clearly huge material to work through in terms of how the erotic is handled, and sometimes appallingly mishandled, in the consulting room. Due to the fear inherent in negotiating this territory, there is a danger that analysts may prefer not to hear (and even, not to speak). If the field valued patient input and was courageous enough to listen, it could be captured more regularly and in more depth without violating the profession's fundamental ethical values. Indeed, doing so would contribute to strengthening those ethical standards. This book offers only one, limited lens from which to understand and explore the erotic transference – and is a success story. I would be delighted if it encouraged other accounts to be published and if it were to spark dialogue and even learning within a field I have come to revere.

I gave a variety of reasons for writing this book earlier. One last reason is that I am trying to seize a sense of permanence from an experience that, despite lasting 5 years, felt so fleeting, intangible and unique. However much we write and whosever voices we include – we are striving to make tangible something that, in the end, cannot be captured; something impossible to translate into cold print. In the words of Orbach (2000, 14): "those twin arcs of therapy, the pentimento and palimpsest, describe a form of great beauty and that beauty, that grace, cannot easily be rendered on the written page". The intense richness of the analytic experience, for either party, cannot possibly be passed to others who were not with us in that 'magical room'. What was truly there will always remain between two people and within them individually – as it should.

The book does mean, though, that something of the experience will always *be* – now that the analysis has ended and even once our memories of it have faded. In this sense, it is a way to 'hold onto the injured bird' while softening the edges of loss as it flies away.

References

Hill, C. (2010) *What Do Patients Want? Psychoanalytic Perspectives from the Couch*. London: Karnac.

Masson, J. (2012) *Final Analysis: The Making and Unmaking of a Psychoanalyst*. E-Published.

Orbach, S. (2000) *The Impossibility of Sex*. New York: Touchstone.

Tessman, L. (2003) *The Analyst's Analyst Within*. London: Analytic Press.

Index

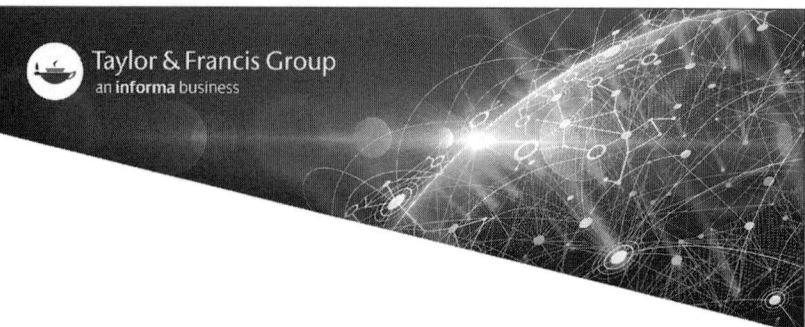
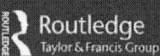
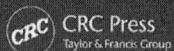

9781032353982